FAST FACTS FOR THE L&D NURSE

Kathryn "Cassie" Giles Groll, DNP, CNM, is a doctorally prepared, Certified Nurse Midwife who is part of a full-scope OB/GYN private practice in New Jersey. She earned her master's degree in nursing and doctorate degree from the University of Medicine and Dentistry of New Jersey. Dr. Groll is licensed in both New Jersey and New York as a Certified Nurse Midwife with prescriptive authority and as an OB/GYN Nurse Practitioner in the state of New York. She has worked as a midwife since 2006 and clinically as an RN in obstetrics in a variety of capacities, including Clinical Instructor of Obstetrics at Columbia University, New York, and High-Risk Women's Health Float Pool at New York-Presbyterian/ Weill Cornell Medical Center, New York City. Dr. Groll is a member of the American College of Nurse Midwives, the Medical History Society of New Jersey, and STTI Honor Society of Nursing. She has served as an advocate for sexual assault victims in Somerset, New Jersey.

FAST FACTS FOR THE L&D NURSE

Labor & Delivery Orientation in a Nutshell

Cassie Giles Groll, DNP, CNM

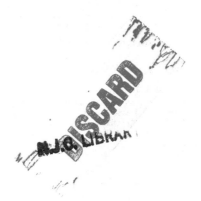

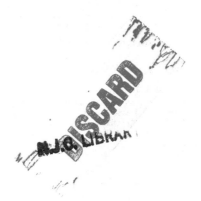

SPRINGER PUBLISHING COMPANY

NEW YORK

Springer Publishing Company, LLC
11 West 42nd Street
New York, NY 10036
www.springerpub.com

Acquisitions Editor: Margaret Zuccarini
Composition: S4Carlisle Publishing Services

ISBN: 978-0-8261-0996-5
E-book ISBN: 978-0-8261-0997-2

14/ 5 4 3

The author and the publisher of this Work have made every effort to use sources believed to be reliable to provide information that is accurate and compatible with the standards generally accepted at the time of publication. Because medical science is continually advancing, our knowledge base continues to expand. Therefore, as new information becomes available, changes in procedures become necessary. We recommend that the reader always consult current research, specific institutional policies, and current drug references before performing any clinical procedure or administering any drug. The author and publisher shall not be liable for any special, consequential, or exemplary damages resulting, in whole or in part, from the readers' use of, or reliance on, the information contained in this book. The publisher has no responsibility for the persistence or accuracy of URLs for external or third-party Internet Web sites referred to in this publication and does not guarantee that any content on such websites is, or will remain, accurate or appropriate.

Library of Congress Cataloging-in-Publication Data

Groll, Cassie Giles.
  Fast facts for the L&D nurse : labor & delivery orientation in a nutshell / Cassie Giles Groll.
    p. ; cm.
  Fast facts for the labor and delivery nurse
  Includes bibliographical references and index.
  ISBN 978-0-8261-0996-5—ISBN 0-8261-0996-9—ISBN 978-0-8261-0997-2 (e-book)
  I. Title. II. Title: Fast facts for the labor and delivery nurse.
    [DNLM: 1. Delivery,   Obstetric—nursing—Handbooks.   2. Labor,   Obstetric—
    Handbooks. WY 49]
  618.2'0231—dc23
                                                                    2012014868

Special discounts on bulk quantities of our books are available to corporations, professional associations, pharmaceutical companies, health care organizations, and other qualifying groups.

If you are interested in a custom book, including chapters from more than one of our titles, we can provide that service as well.

For details, please contact:
Special Sales Department, Springer Publishing Company, LLC
11 West 42nd Street, 15th Floor, New York, NY 10036-8002
Phone: 877-687-7476 or 212-431-4370; Fax: 212-941-7842
Email: sales@springerpub.com

Printed in the United States of America by Gasch Printing.

This book is dedicated to my children, Cooper and Charlotte.

You have both brought me so much happiness and laughter. I cannot imagine my world without you. I live and breathe every second for our next hug. I did not exist until you were born.

And to my husband, Chris, who without his undying support and immense patience, nothing would be possible. I love you.

Contents

Part II: Procedures

Part III: Emergencies

Preface

This book provides basic information pertaining to standard obstetric practices commonly seen in labor and delivery (L&D). Its intent is to reduce the amount of basic questions to coworkers, allowing for more emergent critical questions to be welcomed by more senior staff. This allows new nurses a comfortable independence and confidence in their new environment.

The purpose of this book is not to overwhelm the nurse with information, but to provide a tool that is simple in use and format. It provides clear instructions on what to do, equipment needed, and whom to call in the event of an emergency. It does not take the place of practitioner orders or institutional guidelines.

As the face of medicine changes, the need to use the term *provider* instead of physician or doctor is indicated. Certified nurse midwives are gaining more and more popularity in the obstetric community including private midwifery practices and private physicians' offices. There is much misunderstanding of what exactly a certified nurse midwife does and what the scope of practice is. A certified nurse midwife is a highly skilled, uniquely trained nurse in the field of normal obstetrics and gynecology. He or she can order drugs, deliver babies, do in-office and L&D procedures, as well as assist in surgery. In many hospitals, midwives help train the residents. Most midwives who deliver out of hospitals believe in pain medications for their patients and are highly skilled in emergency situations. They have achieved a postgraduate education, and many of them hold doctorate degrees in the field of nursing or other health-related fields. The regulations and scope of practice vary from state to state, and if you have any questions about what midwives can do on your unit, be sure to ask senior nursing staff or consult your institutional protocols.

A special note to the nurses who use this guide. It is a great responsibility to be an L&D nurse. Although there are days you will forget and will see today as just another day at work, remember it is one of the most amazing days in the life of your patient and she should be met and guided through this process with the same enthusiasm you would want surrounding the birth of your own child. It is also important to remember that as a new life enters this world, he or she should be greeted with love and joyfulness, with profound happiness that he or she is here. You should always be humbled by the fact that it is a privilege to be part of a miracle.

Acknowledgments

I want to express my deepest gratitude to Dr. Elaine Diegmann, CNM, ND, and Dr. Labib Riachi, MD. Elaine, thank you for believing in me and teaching me how to be a midwife, you have given me the most amazing gift, the ability to partake in a miracle. I have been extraordinarily lucky to have been your student. Special thanks to my friend and mentor, Labib, who through the years has been more than generous with his time and expertise. You have taught me more than could ever be found in a textbook. Your guidance and advice have been invaluable, thank you.

This book would not have been possible without my expert panel Dr. Elaine Diegmann, CNM, ND; Dr. Labib Riachi, MD; Dr. Ginette Lange, CNM, PhD; Dr. Joyce Hyatt, CNM, DNP; Ruth Monchek, CNM; and Dr. Russell Hoffman, MD. Their input and immense knowledge were invaluable to this process.

To my friend, Dr. Rachel Behrendt, DNP, I thank you for graciously offering your expertise in proofreading.

And finally, thank you to my husband, Chris, for volunteering to help with the medical illustrations; his talent is beyond words and has made this book visually beautiful.

Thank You

I

General Orientation and Labor and Delivery Overview

In this section, you will find common occurrence on labor and delivery (L&D). It covers definitions, everyday terminology, and common actions with which you should become totally familiar. The section presents a review of medications you may come in contact with on a daily basis including its indication and common dosages. Remember, in the L&D unit you have two patients and your actions must take both patients into account.

MEDICATIONS TO KNOW
- betamethasone (Celestone)
- butorphanol (Stadol)
- calcium gluconate
- carboprost (Hemabate)
- citric acid/sodium citrate (Bicitra)
- dexamethasone
- dinoprostone (Cervidil)
- ephedrine
- erythromycin (erythromycin ophthalmic) ointment
- hydralazine
- indomethacin (Indocin)
- insulin
- labetalol (Trandate)
- lidocaine (Xylocaine)
- magnesium sulfate
- meperidine (Demerol)
- methylergonovine (Methergine)
- misoprostol (Cytotec)
- morphine
- nalbuphine (Nubain)
- naloxone
- nifedipine (Procardia)
- oxytocin (Pitocin)
- promethazine (Phenergan)
- $Rh_o(D)$ immunoglobulin, human (IGIM) (RhoGAM)
- terbutaline
- vitamin K (phytonadione)

ABBREVIATIONS TO LEARN
- AFI—amniotic fluid index
- AFP—alpha fetoprotein
- AROM—artificial rupture of membranes
- CVS—chorionic villa sampling
- DKA—diabetic ketoacidosis

- EDC—estimated date of confinement
- EFW—estimated fetal weight
- FHR—fetal heart rate
- GBS—group B streptococcus
- GC/CT—gonorrhea/*Chlamydia trachomatis*
- GDM—gestational diabetes mellitus
- HBsAg—hepatitis B surface antigen
- ISE—internal scalp electrode
- IUPC—intrauterine pressure catheter
- IUFD—intrauterine fetal demise
- LGA/SGA—large for gestational age/small for gestational age
- LMP—last menstrual period
- MVU—Montevideo units
- NSVD—normal spontaneous vaginal delivery
- PPROM—preterm premature rupture of membranes
- ROM—rupture of membranes
- SROM—spontaneous rupture of membranes
- Toco—tocodynamometer
- UCX—uterine contractions
- U/S—ultrasound
- VBAC—vaginal birth after cesarean section

EQUIPMENT TO LOCATE AND BECOME FAMILIAR WITH

- Compression boots
- Electrosurgery hookup
- Infant pulse oximeter
- Infant warmer
- Infusion pump
- Nitrazine paper
- Pulse oximeter
- Speculum
- Suction hookup
- Tenaculum
- Umbilical cord clamp

Surgical Instruments

- Ring forceps
- T-clamps
- Allis clamps
- Kochers
- Curved Kellys
- Straight Halsteds
- Tube occluding forceps
- Lap sponges
- Bovie tip
- Blades
- Needle holders
- Towel clips
- Scissors
- Forceps
- Scalpels
- Self-Retaining
- Suction tips

AMNIOTIC FLUID

Composed mostly of fetal urine; the volume differs depending on gestation age. It protects and cushions the fetus as well as contributing to GI tract and lung maturity and development.

AMNIOTIC FLUID INDEX (AFI)
- U/S is used to measure AFI
- Abdomen is divided into four quadrants, and largest pocket of fluid in each quadrant is measured
- At least one pocket of fluid needs to be 2 × 2 cm or greater or AFI total >5
- No cord or fetal parts should be present in pocket
- Normal index is between >5 and <25 cm at term

OLIGOHYDRAMNIOS—AFI LESS THAN 5 CM AT TERM
Causes
- ROM
- Genitourinary malformation
- Postdates
- Placental insufficiency

Risks
- Prolonged ROM may lead to infection
- Continued oligohydramnios may cause malformation
- Cord compression leading to fetal hypoxia (nonreassuring tracing)
- Fetal demise

Interventions
- IV fluids for mother
- Antibiotics if preterm
- Induction of labor if term

If patient is in labor, continuous fetal monitoring is possible by amnioinfusion.

POLYHYDRAMNIOS—AFI GREATER THAN 25 CM AT TERM
Causes
- Diabetes mellitus
- Maternal substance abuse
- Tracheoesophageal malformation
- Neural tube defects
- Chromosomal abnormalities
- Twin-to-twin transfusion syndrome

Risks
- Unstable lie of fetus
- Cord prolapse with SROM or AROM

Interventions
- In labor
  - Controlled AROM (needle point) to prevent SROM
  - U/S for fetal lie if patient is in labor
- If preterm,
  - Amnioreduction
  - Indomethacin (Indocin) 25 mg PO q 6 hr $\times$ 48 hr to reduce fetal urine production

ASSESSMENT OF RUPTURE OF MEMBRANES (ROM)
Visual
- Sterile speculum inserted into vagina
- Pooling of fluid noted at fornix of cervix or in vaginal vault
- If unsure, patient should cough to visualize escape of fluid from cervix

Ferning

- Sterile speculum inserted into vagina
- Use cotton swab to obtain fluid
- Smear on slide
- If positive ROM, ferning pattern under microscope will be seen

pH Balance Assessment

- Sterile speculum inserted into vagina
- Touch nitrazine paper to noted fluid
- Normal vaginal pH when pregnant is <4.5
- Amniotic fluid pH is <7.0
- Nitrazine paper/swab changes color to blue at pH <7.0
  - Note: some vaginal infections can cause vaginal pH to reach levels of 7.0 or greater

Amniotic Fluid Protein

- Obtain before vaginal exam
- No speculum necessary
- Insert swab into vagina
- If placental alpha microglobulin-1 is present, test will be positive for ROM
- Follow directions for specific product used by individual institution

SOURCES

Cunningham, G., Leveno, K. J., Bloom, S. L., Hauth, J., Rouse, D., & Spong, C. (2010). *Williams obstetrics* (23rd ed.). New York, NY: McGraw-Hill.

Joseph Hurt, K., Guile, M. W., Bienstock, J. L., Fox, H. E., & Wallach, E. E. (2011). *The Johns Hopkins manual of gynecology and obstetrics* (4th ed.). New York, NY: Lippincott Williams & Wilkins.

Simpson, K. R., & Creehan, P. A. (2008). *Perinatal nursing* (3rd ed.). New York, NY: Lippincott Williams & Wilkins.

Varney, H., Kriebs, J. M., & Gegor, C. L. (2004). *Varney's midwifery* (4th ed.). Sudbury, MA: Jones and Bartlett.

ANTEPARTUM TESTS

INITIAL VISIT 8 TO 12 WEEKS

- U/S for dating
- Pap
- Blood type/Rh factor
- Antibody screen
- GC/CT
- Complete blood count (CBC)
- Syphilis
- HIV
- Hep B
- Rubella titer
- UA
- Hemoglobin electrophoresis
- Cystic fibrosis
- Varicella titers
- Toxoplasmosis
- Cytomegalovirus (CMV)
- Blood glucose (if overweight or history of GDM)

11 TO 13 WEEKS

- First trimester screening (blood work and U/S) for early detection of Down syndrome
- CVS if needed

15 TO 18 WEEKS

- AFP for early detection of neural tube defects
- QUAD if no first trimester screening done or if increased risk for Down syndrome
- Amniocentesis if needed (most commonly done between 16 and 22 weeks)

20 WEEKS

- U/S for fetal anatomy

28 WEEKS

- If patient is Rh neg, RhoGAM should be administered (repeat blood type and Rh factor before administration)
- CBC
- HIV in some states or in high-risk women
- Glucose test

34 TO 36 WEEKS

- GBS (test accurate only for 5 weeks if done at 34 weeks and delivering at 41 weeks; consult with provider if they want to repeat test)
- GC/CT
- Syphilis

SOURCES

Hurt, K. J., Guile, M. W., Bienstock, J. L., Fox, H. E., & Wallach, E. E. (2011). *The Johns Hopkins manual of gynecology and obstetrics* (4th ed.). New York, NY: Lippincott Williams & Wilkins.

Varney, H., Kriebs, J. M., & Gegor, C. L. (2004). *Varney's midwifery* (4th ed.). Sudbury, MA: Jones and Bartlett.

APGAR SCORE

■ A score between 0 and 2 measuring heart rate, muscle tone, respiration rate, color, and reflex of the neonate at 1, 5, and 10 minutes of life

Breathing		
0 Not breathing	1 Slow irregular	2 Crying
Heart Rate		
0 No heartbeat	1 Less than 100	2 Greater than 100
Muscle Tone		
0 Floppy	1 Some tone	2 Active movement
Reflex/Grimace		
0 No response	1 Facial grimace only	2 Pulls away, cries, coughs, or sneezes
Skin Color		
0 Pale blue	1 Body pink, hands and feet blue	2 Entire body is pink

SCORING THE APGAR

■ 1 minute
- Apgar scores are not indicative of future fetal well-being

■ 5 minutes
- 0 to 3 may indicate future neurological problems
- 4 to 6 intermediate scores
- 7 to 10 considered normal scoring range

■ 10 minutes
- should continue to be assessed every 5 minutes if Apgar remains less than 7

Pediatrician should be called in for delivery if

■ Operative delivery
■ Maternal infection or fever
■ Nonreassuring fetal tracing

FAST FACTS in a NUTSHELL

Notify pediatrician immediately if Apgar score is less than 7 at any time.

SOURCES

KidsHealth. (2011). *What is the Apgar score?* Retrieved from http://kidshealth.org/parent/pregnancy_center/q_a/apgar.html#cat32

Varney, H., Kriebs, J. M., & Gegor, C. L. (2004). *Varney's midwifery* (4th ed.). Sudbury, MA: Jones and Bartlett.

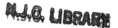

BISHOP SCORE

Scoring system used to determine whether a cervix is inducible or which induction method would be most successful for a vaginal delivery.

Cervix	Bishop score			
	0	1	2	3
Dilation	0 cm	1–2 cm	3–4 cm	>5cm
Effacement	0–30%	40–50%	60–70%	80%
Station	−3	−2	−1/0	+1/+2
Consistency	Firm	Medium	Soft	
Position	Posterior	Mid	Anterior	

From your final total of the bishop score,
- Add 1: for each previous vaginal delivery and/or if patient is preeclamptic
- Subtract 1: for no prior vaginal deliveries if postdates or PPROM
  >4 is considered to be favorable for induction
  <4 would need cervical ripening agent or delaying induction if possible

SOURCES

American College of Obstetricians and Gynecologists. (1999). Induction of labor (Practice bulletin no. 10). In *2008 compendium of selected publications* (p. 603). Washington, DC: Author.

Cunningham, G., Leveno, K. J., Bloom, S. L., Hauth, J., Rouse, D., & Spong, C. (2010). *Williams obstetrics* (23rd ed.). New York, NY: McGraw-Hill.

BREASTFEEDING

Breastfeeding should be initiated immediately after delivery or as soon as possible. It reduces the risk of postpartum hemorrhage (PPH) because it aids in UCX.

POSITIONS
- Cradle hold: across the mother's abdomen, easiest for first-time mothers
- Football hold: infant lies by mother's side supported in her arm
- Side lying: mother is on her side and infant is supported by bed. More difficult position for new mothers

LATCH
- Infant's mouth should be wide open
- Lower lip should make first contact with breast
- Infant should grasp both the areola and the entire nipple (never just the nipple)
- Smacking sounds are indicative of a poor latch

CONTRAINDICATIONS TO BREASTFEEDING
- Mothers who are HIV positive or who have TB
- Mothers who use street drugs

LACTATION DRUG CATEGORIES
- A   Safe—studied on humans
- B   Presumed safe—studied on animals
- C   No studies available
- D   Unsafe—studies have shown adverse effects on infant
- X   Contraindicated—should not be used

SOURCES

Simpson, K. R., & Creehan, P. A. (2008). *Perinatal nursing* (3rd ed.). New York, NY: Lippincott Williams & Wilkins.

Wiessinger, D., West, D., & Pitman, T. (2010). *The womanly art of breastfeeding* (La Leche League International Book) (8th ed.). New York, NY: Ballantine Books.

CERVIX IN LABOR

DILATATION

0 to 10 cm
■ First stage of labor
  • 0 to 3 cm latent phase of labor

Primip average length	6.5 hours
Multip average length	5 hours

  • 4 to 7 cm active phase of labor

Primip average length	4.5 hours
Multip average length	2.5 hours

  • 8 to 10 cm transition phase of labor

Primip average length	3.5 hours
Multip average length	Varies

■ Second stage of labor—10 cm to delivery

Primip average length	up to 3 hours
Multip average length	0 to 30 minutes

■ Third stage of labor—birth to delivery of placenta
  • 0 to 30 minutes

EFFACEMENT
■ Refers to the length of cervix between 0% and 100%

CERVICAL RIPENING

Bishop score can predict success of the induction

Adverse Effects
- Hyperstimulation
- Nonreassuring FHR
- Failed induction

Contraindications
- Prior uterine surgery
- Preterm
- Malposition of fetus, for example, breech or transverse
- Unexplained vaginal bleeding
- Maternal infection or fever of unknown origin

Medications for Cervical Ripening
- dinoprostone (Cervidil) 10 mg PV q 12 hr. Patient must stay in bed for 2 hours after insertion
- dinoprostone (Prepidil) 0.5 mg PV q 6 hr max three doses
- misoprostol (Cytotec) 25 to 50 mcg PV q 3 to 4 hr

Nonpharmacological Cervical Ripening
- Stripping membranes
- Transcervical Foley balloon: inflating a Foley balloon in cervix to dilate

What You Need for Foley Balloon Insertion
- 24 French Foley catheter
- Syringe 30 cc of sterile water
- Sterile gloves
- Speculum
- Tenaculum
- Ring forceps
- Pack of 2 × 2s
- Betadine
- Sterile field

SOURCES

Epocrates. (2011). *Epocrates online*. Retrieved from www.epocrates.com

Hurt, K. J., Guile, M. W., Bienstock, J. L., Fox, H. E., & Wallach, E. E. (2011). *The Johns Hopkins manual of gynecology and obstetrics* (4th ed.). New York, NY: Lippincott Williams & Wilkins.

Simpson, K. R., & Creehan, P. A. (2008). *Perinatal nursing* (3rd ed.). New York, NY: Lippincott Williams & Wilkins.

CESAREAN SECTION (C/S)

CIRCULATING RN'S RESPONSIBILITY
Preparation for C/S
- Admission of patient to L&D
- IV 18G
- Obtaining laboratory reports (type and screen should be drawn within 72 hours of C/S)
- Citric acid/sodium citrate (Bicitra) administration if ordered
- Blood bank type and crossmatch 2 U on standby
- Documenting FHR

In OR
- Verify patient ID, surgery, and physician doing surgery
- Check all equipment (infant warmer, O_2, suction)
- Position for anesthesia
- Apply compression boots
- Insert Foley catheter
- Place electrode pad on thigh
- *First count with scrub tech*
- Drape patient
- Suction hookup
- Electrosurgery hookup
- Notify pediatrician for C/S delivery
- Count after
  - Uterus is closed
  - Fascia closed
  - Skin is closed
- Verify estimated blood loss
- Verify Apgars
- Assist moving patient from OR table to recovery room

General Instruments

Ring forceps	4	Needle holders	4
T-clamps	8	Towel clips	4
Allis clamps	4	Scissors	4
Kochers	4	Forceps	4
Curved Kellys	6	Scalpels	2
Straight Halsteds	6	Self-retaining	6
Tube occluding forceps	5	Suction tips	2
Lap sponges	20		
Bovie tip	1		
Blades	2		
Needles	Depends on surgeon		

Number may vary by institution.

SOURCES

Maternity Center. (2007, April 11). *Maternity Center circulating for cesarean delivery.* Unpublished Procedure Manual, Overlook Hospital Department of Ob/Gyn.

Schaarschmidt, D. (2009, March 9). Charge nurse St. Barnabas Medical Center. Interview.

DATING A PREGNANCY (ASSESSMENT FOR GESTATIONAL AGE)

NAEGELE'S RULE
If patient is sure of LMP,

LMP − 3 Months + 7 Days + 1 Year = EDC

ULTRASOUND
- What is measured
  - Biparietal diameter
  - Head circumference
  - Femoral diaphysis length
  - Abdominal circumference
  - EFW
- Most accurate in first trimester
- Second trimester can be inaccurate by 1 to 2 weeks
- Third trimester can be inaccurate by 2 to 3 weeks

LESS ACCURATE WAYS TO MEASURE (NO CLINICAL DIAGNOSIS SHOULD BE MADE BASED ON FINDINGS)
If patient does not know LMP and no U/S available, you can measure with tape measure or index finger.

Tape Measure
Using centimeter side of tape, measure from pubic symphysis to fundus.

No Tape Measure
Start at umbilicus and measure to top of fundus using the width of your index finger. Start at number 20 and count every finger width as 1 cm. Each finger width or centimeter is equal to 1 gestational week.

GENERAL RULE OF THUMB

- 16 weeks = Halfway between umbilicus and pubic symphysis
- 20 weeks = At umbilicus

FACTORS THAT INFLUENCE UTERINE SIZE IN PREGNANCY

- Full bladder
- AFI
- Fibroids
- Multiple gestations
- Fetal position
- LGA/SGA
- Maternal weight
- Fetal anomalies

SOURCES

American College of Obstetricians and Gynecologists. (2004). Ultrasonography in pregnancy (Practice bulletin no. 58). In *2008 compendium of selected publications* (pp. 859–865). Washington, DC: Author.

Varney, H., Kriebs, J. M., & Gegor, C. L. (2004). *Varney's midwifery* (4th ed.). Sudbury, MA: Jones and Bartlett.

DRUG CLASSIFICATIONS

IN PREGNANCY

A   Controlled studies of pregnant women do not show any adverse effects on fetus.

B   Animal studies have shown no adverse effects on fetus, but no controlled study has been performed on pregnant women.

C   Either there are no studies on animals or pregnant women or animal study showed adverse effect on fetus.

D   Studies on pregnant women did exhibit an adverse effect on fetus. In certain diagnoses, benefits of medication use may outweigh the risks.

X   Contraindicated for women who may attempt or are attempting to become pregnant.

IN LACTATION

L1	Safest	There is no evidence of adverse effects to infant and does not affect the mother's milk supply in large studies
L2	Safer	There is no evidence of adverse effects to infant and does not affect the mother's milk supply in limited studies
L3	Moderately safe	Either no study or effects where minimal with no risk to infant
L4	Possibly hazardous	There is risk to nursing infant or to the production of milk supply
L5	Contraindicated	There is significant risk to infant or to milk production and use should be avoided

SOURCES

Briggs, G. G., Freedman, R. K., & Yaffe, S. J. (2005). *Drugs in pregnancy and lactation* (7th ed.). Philadelphia, PA: Lippincott Williams & Wilkins.

Epocrates. (2011). *Epocrates online.* Retrieved from www.epocrates.com

Perinatology.com. (2011). *Perinatology.com.* Retrieved from www .perinatology.com/exposures/Drugs/FDACategories.htm

ELECTRONIC FETAL MONITORING (EFM)

Three categories for defining and interpreting FHR are as follows:

CATEGORY I
- Normal tracing
  - FHR between 110 and 160
- Moderate variability (beat-to-beat variability is between 6 and 25 bmp)
- Accelerations and early decelerations may or may not be present
- No late or variable decelerations

CATEGORY II

=====*FAST FACTS in a NUTSHELL*

Continuous EFM; NOTIFY physician or midwife.

- Uncertain tracing
  - Marked variability
- Absent variability without recurrent late or variable decelerations
- Tachycardia
- Bradycardia without variability or with minimal variability
- Periodic decelerations
- Recurrent variables without variability or with minimal variability
- Deceleration >2 minutes but <10 minutes
- No acceleration after fetal scalp stimulation

CATEGORY III

=====*FAST FACTS in a NUTSHELL*

ABNORMAL TRACING—CONTACT PHYSICIAN OR MID-WIFE IMMEDIATELY AND NOTIFY SENIOR NURSES.

- Recurrent late or variable decelerations
- Bradycardia
- Sinusoidal pattern

Definitions
- Baseline: FHR between 110 and 160
- Tachycardia: FHR more than 160 (mostly seen with maternal fever)
- Bradycardia: FHR less than 110 (mostly seen in compromised fetus)

Variability
- Minimal: 0 to 5 bpm (may be fetus sleep cycle; continue to monitor)
- Moderate: 6 to 25 bpm (reassuring)
- Marked: greater than 25 bpm (may be a sign of fetal hypoxia)

Acceleration—FHR 15 bpm above baseline for 15 seconds or greater (longer than 10 minutes is change in baseline)

Deceleration—FHR below the baseline
- Early—Nadir of deceleration with peak of contraction (present with pushing or head compression)
- Late—deceleration begins immediately after peak of contraction (recurrent is ominous sign)
- Variable—usually V shaped and may occur at any time. May correlate with cord compression.

Reactive FHR is when two accelerations are noted within a 10-minute period

Sinusoidal—undulating pattern with no baseline or variability able to be appreciated. Usually 3 to 5 cycles/minute. Notify physician or midwife immediately. Seen mostly when a fetus is severely compromised.

Contractions
- Tectonic: resting tone greater than 30 mmHg or firm uterus by palpation

▓ Tachysystole: more than five contractions in a 10-minute period of contraction lasting greater than 90 seconds
▓ Intensity can only be measured with IUPC

Internal Fetal Monitoring (IFM)

ISE—electrode that is attached to fetal scalp. Most accurate way to assess FHR. Membranes must be ruptured and patient must be 2 to 3 cm dilated

What You Need

▓ Sterile gloves
▓ ISE lead and connecting wire
▓ Tape (to tape lead to patient's leg)
▓ Amnihook if needed for AROM
▓ FHR will sound like a "ping" when working appropriately

IUPC—catheter is inserted and lies next to fetus to measure pressure of contractions within the uterus. This is the only way to document accurate uterine resting tone and intensity. Membranes must be ruptured and patient must be 2 to 3 cm dilated.

What You Need

▓ Sterile gloves
▓ IUPC lead and connecting wire
▓ Tape (to tape lead to patient's leg)
▓ After first contraction, zero out the IUPC to assess accurate resting tone
▓ Amnihook if needed for AROM

Documentation

▓ Baseline EHR
▓ Variability
▓ Acceleration and decelerations present
▓ Contractions
▓ EFM versus ISE
▓ Toco versus IUPC
▓ Notification of physician or midwife
▓ Intervention and outcome

Intrauterine Resuscitation
Nonreassuring Tracing
- Stop induction agent, for example, oxytocin (Pitocin) or remove dinoprostone (Cervidil)
- Remove dinoprostone (Cervidil)
- Give 10 L/minute of O_2 through facemask
- Increase IV fluids
- Change maternal position
- Anticipate possible amnioinfusion
- Notify physician or midwife

Tachysystole
- Stop induction agent, for example, oxytocin (Pitocin) or remove dinoprostone (Cervidil)
- Remove dinoprostone (Cervidil)
- Increase IV fluids
- Anticipate tocolytics to be given (e.g., Terbutaline 0.25 mg SQ)
- Notify physician or midwife

Hypotension (Maternal)
- Lay patient flat
- Increase IV fluids
- Anticipate ephedrine 5 to 10 mg IV push (not for RN administration)
- Notify anesthetist and physician or midwife

SOURCES
American College of Obstetricians and Gynecologists. (2009). Intrapartum fetal heart rate monitoring: Nomenclature, interpretation, and general management principles (Practice bulletin no. 106). In *2009 compendium of selected publications* (pp. 192–202). Washington, DC: Author.

Hurt, K. J., Guile, M. W., Bienstock, J. L., Fox, H. E., & Wallach, E. E. (2011). *The Johns Hopkins manual of gynecology and obstetrics* (4th ed.). New York, NY: Lippincott Williams & Wilkins.

Simpson, K. R., & Creehan, P. A. (2008). *Perinatal nursing* (3rd ed.). New York, NY: Lippincott Williams & Wilkins.

EMERGENCY DRUGS

Indication	Drug name—generic (trade)	Dosage, route, and frequency	Comments/cautions
Preterm labor			
Corticosteroids (for fetal lung maturity)			
	betamethasone (Celestone)	12 mg IM q 12 hr × 2 doses	
	dexamethasone	6 mg IM q 12 hr × 4 doses	
Tocolytics (to try and stop labor)			
	indomethacin (Indocin)	50–100 mg PO at first dose, then 25–50 mg PO q 4–6 hr	Do not give if oligohydramnios
	nifedipine (Procardia)	10–20 mg PO q 6 hr	
	terbutaline	0.25 mg SQ q 20–30 min PRN	May cause maternal tachycardia
	magnesium sulfate	Loading dose: 4–6 g IV, then 2–4 g IV/hr	Serum magnesium (Mg) level should be drawn q 6 hr. Levels should be between 6 and 8 mg/dl Levels 8–10 mg/dl = decrease deep tendon reflexes Levels 13–15 mg/dl = respiratory distress Levels >15 mg/dl = cardiac arrest Monitor I&O Manage IV drip so no more than 125 ml/hr infuses ANTIDOTE: calcium gluconate 1 g IV over 3 min

(continues)

(continued)

Indication	Drug name—generic (trade)	Dosage, route, and frequency	Comments/cautions
Postpartum hemorrhage			
	oxytocin (Pitocin)	10 IU/ml IM or 40 units IV	Should have drug in room at every delivery
	methylergonovine (Methergine)	0.2 mg IM q 2–4 hr	Do not give hypertension (HTN)/preeclamptic patients Keep in refrigerator
	carboprost (Hemabate)	250 mcg IM q 15–90 min; maximum 8 doses	Do not give with history of asthma
	misoprostel (Cytotec)	800–1,000 mcg rectal	
Preeclampsia			
	magnesium sulfate	Loading dose: 4–6 g IV, then 2–4 g IV/hr	Serum magnesium (Mg) level should be drawn q 6 hr. Levels should be between 6 and 8 mg/dl Levels 8–10 mg/dl = decrease deep tendon reflexes Levels 13–15 mg/dl = respiratory distress Levels >15 mg/dl = cardiac arrest Monitor I&O Manage IV drip so no more than 125 ml/hr infuses ANTIDOTE: calcium gluconate 1 g IV over 3 min

(continues)

(continued)

Indication	Drug name— generic (trade)	Dosage, route, and frequency	Comments/cautions
	labetalol (Trandate)	20 mg IV push then increase dose at 10 min intervals to 20, 40, 80 mg, for max 300 mg/24 hr	NOT FOR RN ADMINISTRATION
	hydralazine	5 mg IV bolus q 20 min until 20 mg PRN	
Opioid-addicted mother (for nonresponsive or low Apgar neonate)			
	nalozone	0.1 mg/kg IV, IM, or SQ, q 2–3 min PRN	Pediatrician should be at delivery

═══════════════════════════════ *FAST FACTS in a NUTSHELL*

ANTIDOTE [for hypermagnesemia]: calcium gluconate 1 g IV over 3 minutes; should be in room if MgSO$_4$ is infusing.

SOURCES

American College of Obstetricians and Gynecologists. (2006). Postpartum hemorrhage (Practice bulletin no. 108). In *2008 compendium of selected publications* (pp. 1039–1047). Washington, DC: Author.

Drug information online. (2011). *Drugs.com.* Retrieved from www.drugs.com

Epocrates. (2011). *Epocrates online.* Retrieved from www.epocrates.com

Hurt, K. J., Guile, M. W., Bienstock, J. L., Fox, H. E., & Wallach, E. E. (2011). *The Johns Hopkins manual of gynecology and obstetrics* (4th ed.). New York, NY: Lippincott Williams & Wilkins.

Simpson, K. R., & Creehan, P. A. (2008). *Perinatal nursing* (3rd ed.). New York, NY: Lippincott Williams & Wilkins.

FETAL DEMISE (IUFD)

Cardiac activity is not noted by real-time U/S after 20 weeks, often referred to as stillborn.

If possible, take infant warmer out of room before patient is admitted to room. Place a sign (often a picture) indicating that there is a fetal demise so that other personnel on the unit are aware.

WHAT TO DO
- Proceed as with induction
- Admit to L&D
- IV access
- Admission labs
- Toco (ONLY)
- Vital signs (VS)
- Patient history

Depending on Bishop score and gestational age, the determination of appropriate medication should be ordered by physician or midwife.

MOST OFTEN ORDERED INDUCTION AGENTS
- misoprostol (Cytotec)
- oxytocin (Pitocin)

WHAT TO EXPECT
- Delivery is often quick once patient has dilated
- Placenta delivery may take longer than 30 minutes
- Be prepared, be sensitive, and be professional

WHAT TO DO

- Wrap the baby and offer to mother
- Save baby hat, take photos and footprints and put all in memory box
- Give supportive care as needed
- Contact social worker and/or pastoral care (as appropriate)

FAST FACTS in a NUTSHELL

The organization *Now I Lay Me Down To Sleep* provides families with free professional photography sessions. If a photographer is available in your area, the family should be informed and given the option.

SOURCES

Maternity Center. (2010, March 10). *Maternity Center induction of labor for fetal demise/nonviable fetus.* Unpublished Procedure Manual, Overlook Hospital Department of Ob/Gyn.

Now I lay me down to sleep. (2011). Retrieved from www .nowilaymedowntosleep.org

FETAL KICK COUNTS

Used to assess the well-being of the fetus. Test is subjective and performed by the mother.

PROCESS FOR CONDUCTING THE TEST
- Done after 28 weeks' gestation
- Have the mother lie on her left side
- Instruct her to count the number of kicks or movements she feels within 2 hours

INTERPRETATION OF THE TEST
- Reassuring: If more than 10 movements are counted.
- Patient should call her provider immediately or come to L&D for assessment, if fewer than 10 are counted or if no movements are felt.
- If patient states she has felt no fetal movement for 24 hours, she should be seen immediately.

SOURCES
American College of Obstetricians and Gynecologists. (2011). *ACOG education pamphlet AP098-special tests for monitoring fetal health*. Retrieved from www.acog.org/publications/patient_education/bp098.cfm
Simpson, K. R., & Creehan, P. A. (2008). *Perinatal nursing* (3rd ed.). New York, NY: Lippincott Williams & Wilkins.

GESTATIONAL DIABETES MELLITUS (GDM)

Usually diagnosed between 16 and 28 weeks of pregnancy depending on maternal risk factor

MATERNAL COMPLICATIONS
- DKA
- Preeclampsia
- Preterm labor and delivery

FETAL COMPLICATIONS
- Congenital malformation
- Polyhydramnios
- Macrosomia
- Intrauterine growth restriction (IUGR)
- Fetal demise
- Shoulder dystocia
- Neonatal hypoglycemia

MANAGEMENT
- Patients may be induced between 39 and 40 weeks
- Patients with EFW greater than the 4,500 g—C/S delivery is indicated
- Prepare room for shoulder dystocia for anticipated NSVD

MANAGEMENT ON L&D
- Normal saline IV
- Finger stick: q hour until stable (between 70 and 110 mg/dl)
  - q 2 hr until delivery
- Notify MD if glucose is <60 or >150 mg/dl
- Monitor hourly I&Os
- Continuous fetal monitoring

WHAT YOU NEED FOR AN INSULIN DRIP
(USUALLY NOT FOR PATIENTS WHO HAVE TYPE 2 OR GDM)

- Infusion pump
- Insulin is ALWAYS intravenous piggy back (IVPB) to primary IV of normal saline
- Prime IV tubing with at least 50 ml of insulin solution before starting infusion
- Insulin drip is 100 U of regular insulin in 100 ml of normal saline
- Follow orders and institutional protocol for rate
- Discontinue drip at time of delivery

HYPOGLYCEMIA CLINICAL PRESENTATION

- Blood sugar <60 mg/dl
- Nausea
- Headache
- Diaphoresis
- Visual changes
- Weakness
- Confusion

WHAT TO DO FOR HYPOGLYCEMIA

- Notify MD immediately
- If no IV, give 4 ounces of juice
- If you have an IV, start D5NS at 12 ml/hr
- Repeat finger stick q 15 min until BS above 70 mg/dl

DIABETIC KETOACIDOSIS (DKA)

Not enough circulating insulin in the body to metabolize glucose

Clinical Presentation

- Abdominal pain
- Nausea
- Vomiting
- Hypotension
- Tachypnea
- Confusion
- Lethargy
- Sweet-smelling breath

WHAT TO DO

- Call physician STAT
- Call anesthetist STAT
- EKG STAT
- Blood gases STAT (may need to call respiratory to obtain)
- Labs: CMP, acetone, and ketone bodies STAT and then q 1 to 2 hr
- 18G IV started with normal saline bolus 1 L over 30 minutes
- Give O_2 8 to 10 L/min through facemask
- EFM continuous
- Pulse oximetry continuous
- Anticipate: Intubation
  - Insulin infusion as per physician orders
  - Sodium bicarbonate as ordered if pH is <7.1
- Monitor for signs of pulmonary edema
  - Hypovolemia
  - Cerebral edema

=== *FAST FACTS in a NUTSHELL*

Antenatal steroids and tocolytics can cause or worsen DKA.

SOURCES

American College of Obstetricians and Gynecologists. (2005). Pregestational diabetes mellitus (Practice bulletin no. 60). In *2008 compendium of selected publications* (pp. 868–877). Washington, DC: Author.

Hurt, K. J., Guile, M. W., Bienstock, J. L., Fox, H. E., & Wallach, E. E. (2011). *The Johns Hopkins manual of gynecology and obstetrics* (4th ed.). New York, NY: Lippincott Williams & Wilkins.

Maternity Center. (2008, June 11). *Maternity Center diabetic patient.* Unpublished Procedure Manual, Overlook Hospital Department of Ob/Gyn.

Simpson, K. R., & Creehan, P. A. (2008). *Perinatal nursing* (3rd ed.). New York, NY: Lippincott Williams & Wilkins.

GROUP B STREPTOCOCCUS (GBS)

A gram-positive bacterium that colonizes in the vagina, urethra, and/or rectum and can cause premature birth/premature rupture of membranes (PROM), sepsis, pneumonia, and meningitis. Swab should be obtained at 35 to 37 weeks. If results were negative and patient delivers 5 weeks after initial GBS screening, consider obtaining another swab.

2010 GUIDELINES

Intrapartum (IP) GBS prophylaxis indicated	IP GBS prophylaxis not indicated
- Previous infant with invasive GBS disease	- Colonization with GBS during a previous pregnancy (unless an indication for GBS prophylaxis is present for current pregnancy)
- GBS bacteriuria during any trimester of the current pregnancy	- GBS bacteriuria during previous pregnancy (unless an indication for GBS prophylaxis is present for current pregnancy)
- Positive GBS vaginal-rectal screening culture in late gestation during current pregnancy	- Negative vaginal and rectal GBS screening culture in late gestation during the current pregnancy, regardless of IP risk factors
- Unknown GBS status at the onset of labor (culture not done, incomplete, or results unknown) and any of the following: Delivery at <37 wk gestation — Amniotic membrane rupture ≥18 hr — IP temperature ≥38°C — IP NAAT positive for GBS	- Cesarean delivery performed before onset of labor on a woman with intact amniotic membranes, regardless of GBS colonization status or gestational age

Abbreviation: NAAT, nucleic acid amplification tests.

From Centers for Disease Control and Prevention (2010).

TREATMENT IN PRETERM LABOR

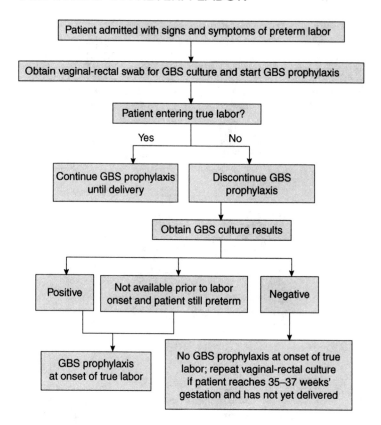

From Centers for Disease Control and Prevention (2010).

If patient has PPROM, swab and treat for 48 hours.

TREATMENT IN LABOR

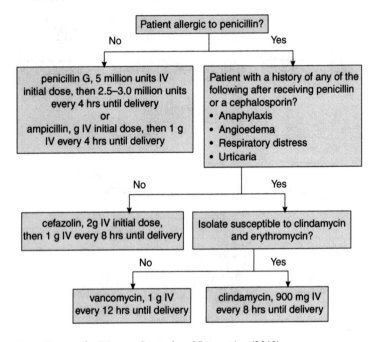

From Centers for Disease Control and Prevention (2010).

SOURCES

Centers for Disease Control and Prevention. (2010). Prevention of perinatal group B Streptococcal disease. *Morbidity and Mortality Weekly Report, 59*(RR10), 1–32.

Centers for Disease Control and Prevention. (2011). *Prevention of perinatal group B streptococcal disease.* Retrieved from www.cdc.gov/groupbstrep/clinicians/obstetric-providers.html#algorithms

Scharf, S., Verani, J., & McGee, L. (2010). Prevention of perinatal group B streptococcal disease. *Morbidity and Mortality Weekly Report, 59*(RR10), 1–32.

Varney, H., Kriebs, J. M., & Gegor, C. L. (2004). *Varney's midwifery* (4th ed.). Sudbury, MA: Jones and Bartlett.

LABOR PROGRESSION

STAGES OF LABOR

■ First stage of labor
  • 0 to 3 cm latent phase of labor

Primip average length	6.5 hours
Multip average length	5 hours

  • 4 to 7 cm active phase of labor

Primip average length	4.5 hours
Multip average length	2.5 hours

  • 8 to 10 cm transition phase of labor

Primip average length	3.5 hours
Multip average length	varies

  • Second stage of labor—10 cm to delivery

Primip average length	up to 3 hours
Multip average length	0 to 3 minutes

■ Third stage of labor—birth to delivery of placenta
  • 0 to 30 minutes

PHASES OF LABOR

■ Latent phase: beginning of regular UCX until cervix is dilated 3 to 4 cm
■ Active phase: cervix is 3 to 4 cm dilated until cervix is 10 cm (fully dilated)
■ Transitional phase: the end of the first stage of labor *transitioning* into the second stage of labor

DYSTOCIA OF LABOR

- Premature rupture of membranes: ROM prior to the onset of labor
- Arrest of labor (failure of descent or failure to progress): at least 4 cm, adequate UCX (200 to 225 MVU) and no cervical dilatation in 4 hours

SOURCES

American College of Obstetricians and Gynecologists. (2003). Dystocia and augmentation of labor (Practice bulletin no. 49). In *2008 compendium of selected publications* (pp. 802–811). Washington, DC: Author.

Cunningham, G., Leveno, K. J., Bloom, S. L., Hauth, J., Rouse, D., & Spong, C. (2010). *Williams obstetrics* (23rd ed). New York, NY: McGraw-Hill.

Hurt, K. J., Guile, M. W., Bienstock, J. L., Fox, H. E., & Wallach, E. E. (2011). *The Johns Hopkins manual of gynecology and obstetrics* (4th ed.). New York, NY: Lippincott Williams & Wilkins.

Simpson, K. R., & Creehan, P. A. (2008). *Perinatal nursing* (3rd ed.). New York, NY: Lippincott Williams & Wilkins.

LABS

SKELETONS/FISHBONES

The correct format to represent your laboratory values in a paper chart.

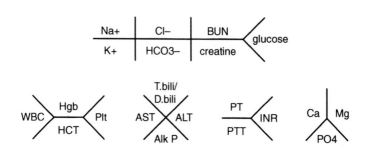

═══*FAST FACTS in a NUTSHELL*

If at any time a patient may need to have a C/S, blood bank should be called and 2 units should be crossmatched and readily available. Refrigerator in unit should also have O neg (emergency release) blood and should be checked to ensure it is not expired at the beginning of every shift.

ABDOMINAL TRAUMA

- Type and screen
- Antibody screen
- Crossmatch (if patient may need C/S)
- CBC
- KB
- Coagulation profile
- Toxicology

ABRUPTIO PLACENTAE
- CBC
- Type and screen
- PT/PTT
- Fibrinogen
- Fibrin split products
- Toxicology

ADMISSION LABS TO L&D
- CBC
- Urine dipstick
- Blood type and Rh
- Antibody screen
- RPR: if not in prenatal record
- HBsAg: if not in prenatal record
- Rubella: if not in prenatal record

AMNIOTIC FLUID EMBOLISM
- Type and screen (if admission labs not obtained)
- Arterial blood gases
- Serum electrolytes
- CMP
- Coagulation profile
- CBC

PREECLAMPSIA
- CBC
- Liver function panel
- Kidney function panel
- PT/PTT
- Fibrinogen
- Urine dipstick/urinalysis
- 24-hour urine collection

SOURCES

American College of Obstetricians and Gynecologists. (2002). Diagnosis and management of preeclampsia and eclampsia (Practice bulletin no. 33). In *2008 compendium of selected publications* (pp. 717–725). Washington, DC: Author.

Cunningham, G., Leveno, K. J., Bloom, S. L., Hauth, J., Rouse, D., & Spong, C. (2010). *Williams obstetrics* (23rd ed.). New York, NY: McGraw-Hill.

Curran, C. A. (2003). Intrapartum emergencies. *Journal of Obstetric, Gynecologic, & Neonatal Nursing, 32,* 802–813. doi:10.1177/0884217503258425

Hurt, K. J., Guile, M. W., Bienstock, J. L., Fox, H. E., & Wallach, E. E. (2011). *The Johns Hopkins manual of gynecology and obstetrics* (4th ed.). New York, NY: Lippincott Williams & Wilkins.

MAGNESIUM SULFATE (MgSO$_4$)

Used for preeclampsia/eclampsia and preterm labor (PTL). The drug affects the central nervous system (CNS) and functions as a smooth muscle relaxer and anticonvulsant.

In the use of magnesium sulfate for preeclampsia/eclampsia, the drug is given as an anticonvulsant, not for hypertension. A side effect is a decrease in blood pressure (BP), but this may be temporary and have a rebound effect. Continue to monitor BP and notify practitioner if it exceeds perimeters.

Magnesium sulfate will not work for PTL if the patient is in active labor.

SIDE EFFECTS
- Flushing
- Muscle weakness
- Blurred vision
- Headache
- Lethargy
- Nausea/vomiting
- Bradycardia
- Respiratory depression

CONTRAINDICATIONS
- Respiratory depression
- Systolic BP <110
- Heart block
- Myasthenia gravis

ADMINISTRATION
- magnesium sulfate
  - Loading dose 4 to 6 g IV
  - Maintenance 2 to 4 g IV/hr
  - Serum Mg level should be drawn q 6 hr.
  - Levels should be between 6 and 8 mg/dl

■ Serum Mg levels
  • 6 to 8 mg/dl therapeutic
  • 8 to 10 mg/dl decrease deep tendon reflexes
  • 13 to 15 mg/dl respiratory distress
  • >15 mg/dl cardiac arrest

Monitor I&Os and IV fluid needs to be managed so no more than 125 ml/hr of total IV fluids is infusing

═══════════════════════════════════*FAST FACTS in a NUTSHELL*

ANTIDOTE [to hypermagnesemia]: calcium gluconate 1 g IV over 3 minutes; should be in room if MgSO$_4$ is infusing.

SOURCES

American College of Obstetricians and Gynecologists. (2002a). Diagnosis and management of preeclampsia and eclampsia (Practice bulletin no. 33). In *2008 compendium of selected publications* (pp. 717–725). Washington, DC: Author.

American College of Obstetricians and Gynecologists. (2002b). Management of preterm labor (Practice bulletin no. 43). In *2008 compendium of selected publications* (pp. 765–773). Washington, DC: Author.

Drug Information Online. (2011). *Drugs.com*. Retrieved from www.drugs.com

Epocrates. (2011). *Epocrates online*. Retrieved from www.epocrates.com

MONTEVIDEO UNITS (MVU)

Measures the intensity of UCX and diagnoses their adequacy for labor. Can be done only when an IUPC is in place.

WHAT YOU NEED FOR IUPC PLACEMENT
- Amnihook if needed for AROM
- Sterile gloves
- IUPC lead and connecting wire
- Tape (to tape lead to patient's leg)
- After first contraction, zero out the IUPC to assess accurate resting tone
- Amnihook if needed for AROM

TO CALCULATE MVU
Take the contraction strength of each contraction occurring within a 10-minute period and add the intensity together.

TO CALCULATE INTENSITY OF UCX
Take the baseline uterine pressure and subtract it from the peak height of the contraction.

   Example intensity calculation: Uterine resting tone is at 20 mmHg; the peak of that UCX is 100 mmHg.

100 mmHg	UCX intensity = 80 mmHg
−20 mmHg	
80 mmHg	

Example MVU calculation: Patient has 3 UCX in 10 minutes each with the below intensity.

80 mmHg	MVU=225
75 mmHg	
+70 mmHg	
225 mmHg	

Adequate contracts are measured above 200 mmHg MVU.

SOURCES

Cunningham, G., Leveno, K. J., Bloom, S. L., Hauth, J., Rouse, D., & Spong, C. (2010). *Williams obstetrics* (23rd ed.). New York, NY: McGraw-Hill.

Maternity Center. (2010, June 9). *Maternity Center: Intrauterine pressure catheter.* Unpublished Procedure Manual, Overlook Hospital Department of Ob/Gyn.

MULTIPLE GESTATIONS

A pregnancy where more than one fetus is conceived at the same time. Can be spontaneous or because of infertility treatment. Most facilities allow cephalic/cephalic to try NSVD; however, if cephalic/breech a C/S is usually performed. Most vaginal twins are delivered in the OR.

RISKS/COMPLICATIONS
- PTL/delivery
- IUGR
- Preeclampsia
- Postpartum hemorrhage
- Gestational diabetes
- Twin-to-twin transfusion
- Cord accident (monochromic/monoamniotic)
- Increase occurrence of C/S
- Placental abnormalities

TYPES OF MULTIPLE GESTATIONS

	Approximate occurrence (%)	Placenta	Amniotic sac
Dizygotic dichorionic/ diamnionic (fraternal)	75	2	2
Monozygotic (identical)	25	Varies depending on time of cleavage	Varies depending on time of cleavage
Dichorionic/ diamnionic monozygotic	8	2	2
Monochorionic/ diamnionic	17	1 fused	2
Monochorionic/ monoamnionic	<1	1	1

SOURCES

Hurt, K. J., Guile, M. W., Bienstock, J. L., Fox, H. E., & Wallach, E. E. (2011). *The Johns Hopkins manual of gynecology and obstetrics* (4th ed.). New York, NY: Lippincott Williams & Wilkins.

Varney, H., Kriebs, J. M., & Gegor, C. L. (2004). *Varney's midwifery* (4th ed.). Sudbury, MA: Jones and Bartlett.

NEWBORN

If possible, always place the baby on the mother immediately after delivery. Infant can be cleaned, wrapped in a blanket or skin-to-skin, VS taken, and ID bands placed, all while on the mother's chest.

ROOM SETUP

Access to all the mother's antenatal blood work

- Warmer
- Blankets
- Oxygen
- Suction
- Diaper
- Infant hat
- Laryngoscope
- Umbilical cord clamp
- Scissors
- Thermometer
- Infant pulsometer
- Erythromycin (erythromycin ophthalmic) ointment 0.5% (*administered in newborn's eyes for prophylaxis against GC/CT*)
- Vitamin K (phytonadione) 1 mg IM × 1 dose (*administered in newborns for prophylaxis of classic hemorrhagic disease*)

WHAT TO DO

- Assess the newborn (if at any point the Apgars are less than 7, notify pediatrician STAT)
- Place ID bands on mother and infant
- Document time of birth and placenta delivery
- Obtain cord blood
- Assist mother in breastfeeding

SOURCES

Simpson, K. R., & Creehan, P. A. (2008). *Perinatal nursing* (3rd ed.). New York, NY: Lippincott Williams & Wilkins.

Varney, H., Kriebs, J. M., & Gegor, C. L. (2004). *Varney's midwifery* (4th ed.). Sudbury, MA: Jones and Bartlett.

PAIN MANAGEMENT

DISTRACTION METHODS
- Guided imagery
- Music
- Focal points
- Relaxation techniques
- Breathing techniques

POSITIONS THAT MOST COMMONLY RELIEVE PRESSURE AND DISCOMFORT
- Walking
- Swaying
- Sitting on toilet
- Leaning over back of bed (raise the back hospital bed to upright position; mother kneels on bed)
- Squatting
- Lying on her side
- Sitting on a birthing ball

INTERVENTIONS TO RELIEVE BACK PAIN
- Ice packs to lower back
- Getting into shower with water directed to lower back
- Getting into bathtub
- Counter pressure (someone places their fists on mother's lower back and presses hard during contraction)

MOST COMMON IV MEDICATION
Phenergan is often given to potentiate the effects of pain medication; however, it is extremely caustic and should be used with caution and be administered only in a diluted solution to prevent phlebitis or other vascular injury.

Caution should be taken when administering IV pain medication. IV pain medication should be administered only if the delivery time is anticipated to be more than 4 hours from the time of administration to avoid possible respiratory depression in the neonate.

Patient should not be ambulatory after medication is administered.

nalbuphine (Nubain)	5–10 mg	q 4 hr PRN
morphine	1–2 mg	q 4 hr PRN
butorphanol (Stadol)	1–2 mg	q 4 hr PRN
meperidine (Demerol)	25–50 mg	q 4 hr PRN
promethazine (Phenergan) (also used for nausea in labor)	12.5–25 mg	q 4 hr PRN

Side Effects
- Lethargy
- Respiratory depression for mother and neonate
- Disorientation
- Pruritus
- Hypotension

LOCAL ANESTHESIA
Lidocaine injection lasts approximately 20 to 40 minutes and gives relief for the cutting episiotomies and repairing vaginal laceration. Pudendal block allows for pain relief during a vaginal delivery due to numbing effects of lidocaine being injected into the pudendal nerve space.

Side Effects
- Cardiac arrhythmia
- Hematoma
- Infection at injection site

EPIDURAL/COMBINED SPINAL EPIDURAL

Catheter placed into dural space, anesthesia medications are given through catheter and block the nerve impulses from the lower spinal segments. Provides most comprehensive pain relief for delivery.

Side Effects

- Pruritus
- Hypotension
- Headache
- Fetal bradycardia
- Possible increase in length of labor
- Urinary retention

SOURCES

Cunningham, G., Leveno, K. J., Bloom, S. L., Hauth, J., Rouse, D., & Spong, C. (2010). *Williams obstetrics* (23rd ed.). New York, NY: McGraw-Hill.

Simpson, K. R., & Creehan, P. A. (2008). *Perinatal nursing* (3rd ed.). New York, NY: Lippincott Williams & Wilkins.

PITOCIN

The synthetic hormone of oxytocin. It is used for labor induction and augmentation. It is also used in the immediate postpartum period to reduce PPH by causing the uterus to contract.

Fetal heart rate and uterine contractions MUST be monitored when administering Pitocin.

SIDE EFFECTS
- Uterine hypertonicity
- Uterine rupture
- Abruptio placentae
- Arrhythmias
- Hypertension
- Fetal distress
- Hyperbilirubinemia of neonate
- Nausea
- Vomiting

CONTRAINDICATIONS
- Fetal malpresentation
- Fetal distress
- MVU above 200 without progression of cervical dilatation
- Adequate contraction pattern already established
- Any contraindication for vaginal delivery
- Classical or fundal prior uterine incision
- Use with extreme caution and at a low dose for VBACs. ONLY to be used with women who have had a lower segment transverse uterine incision documented and in chart (Consult policy and procedure manual for individual institution protocol)

WHAT YOU NEED
- Pitocin
- IV pump
- Main IV fluid already infusing
- IV tubing
- Orders for administration
- Toco and EFM or IUPC and ISE in place

ADMINISTRATION
- If at any time infusion is being discontinued for fetal distress ordering, practitioner should be notified.
- Must have written order from midwife or physician to start Pitocin with strict adherence to hospital protocol.
- Must have adequate monitoring before administration to show inadequate contraction patterns and stability of FHR.

Labor Induction/Augmentation
Most Common Titration
   30 U/500 ml LR = 60 mU/ml

Example
   2 mU/min = 2 ml/hr

IVPB
Start
   1 to 2 mU/min

Increase
   1 to 2 mU/min every 20 to 30 min PRN

Maximum Dose
   20 mU/min

Postpartum
IV
- After delivery of placenta,
  - 20 mU/L IV at 125 ml/hr
- For increased bleeding,
  - 40 mU/L IV may infuse faster than 125 ml/hr depending on institutional protocol

IM
- 10 U IM × 1 dose after the delivery of the placenta
- If heavy bleeding continues, start IV, give 500 cc bolus of LR (if bolus is not contraindicated) and prepare to administer Methergine or Hemabate.

═══════════════════════*FAST FACTS in a NUTSHELL*

ANTIDOTE (for tachysystole): Terbutaline 0.25 mg SC q 20 min PRN.

SOURCES

Epocrates. (2011). *Epocrates online.* Retrieved from www.epocrates.com

Maternity Center. (2010, March 10). *Maternity Center oxytocin administration and augmentation of labor.* Unpublished Procedure Manual, Overlook Hospital Department of Ob/Gyn.

Simpson, K. R., & Creehan, P. A. (2008). *Perinatal nursing* (3rd ed.). New York, NY: Lippincott Williams & Wilkins.

RhoGAM

- Only for Rh-neg women
- Anti-D immunoglobulin (human) is given to women during their pregnancy if they are Rh neg. It stops antibody formation against the fetus if the fetus is Rh pos. It prevents newborn hemolytic disease and protects future pregnancies against alloimmunization.
- RhoGAM 300 mcg IM

ROUTINE ADMINISTRATION

- 26 to 28 weeks' gestational age
- Within 72 hours after delivery (if the infant is Rh pos)

OTHER INDICATIONS FOR ADMINISTRATION

- Maternal hx of blood transfusion
- Hx of previous newborns needing blood transfusions
- Ectopic pregnancy
- Elective or spontaneous abortion
- CVS or amniocentesis
- Fetal demise
- Second and/or third trimester bleeding
- Abdominal trauma

CONTRAINDICATED

- Rh-pos women
- Newborn blood type is Rh neg

SOURCES

American College of Obstetricians and Gynecologists. (1999). Prevention of Rh D Alloimmunization (Practice bulletin no. 4). In *2008 compendium of selected publications* (pp. 573–580). Washington, DC: Author.

RhoGAM. (2011). Retrieved from www.rhogam.com/Professional/Pages/default.aspx

SURGICAL INSTRUMENTS

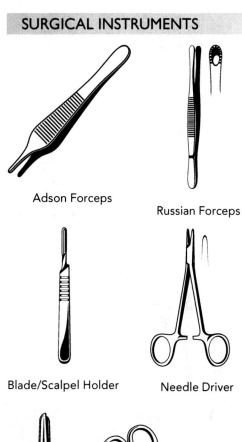

Adson Forceps

Russian Forceps

Debakey Forceps

Blade/Scalpel Holder

Needle Driver

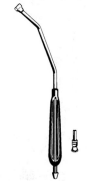

Yankauer Suction

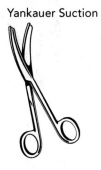

Mayo Scissors

Bandage Scissors

Curved Mayo

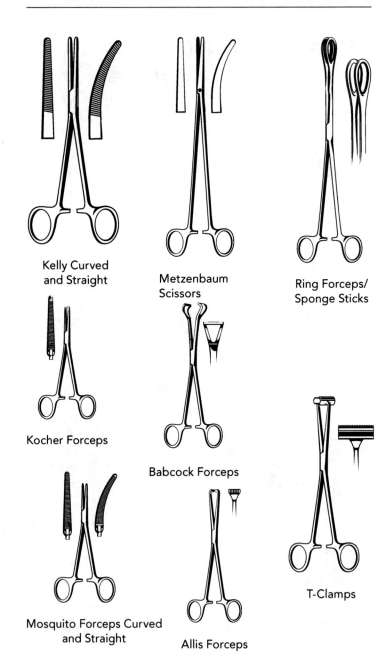

Kelly Curved
and Straight

Metzenbaum
Scissors

Ring Forceps/
Sponge Sticks

Kocher Forceps

Babcock Forceps

T-Clamps

Mosquito Forceps Curved
and Straight

Allis Forceps

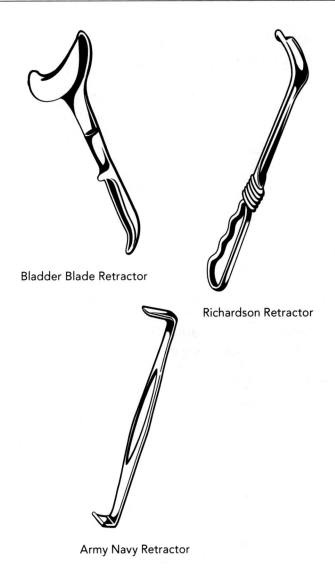

Bladder Blade Retractor

Richardson Retractor

Army Navy Retractor

SOURCE
Groll, C. (2011). *Surgical instrument illustrations.* Cranford, NJ.

VAGINAL BIRTH AFTER CESAREAN SECTION (VBAC)

Previous OR report should be in chart stating low transverse uterine incision

CONTRAINDICATIONS
- Previous classical incision, T-scar on uterus, fundal incision
- Previous uterine rupture
- Macrosomic fetus
- Multiple gestations
- Any contraindication to a vaginal delivery
- Less than 18 months since last C/S
- Cytotec
- The number of prior deliveries by low transverse C/S followed by a vaginal delivery is currently under debate; follow institutional guidelines

Epidural and low-dose Pitocin are NOT contraindicated

ADVERSE OUTCOMES
- Uterine rupture 1%
- Failed attempt at vaginal delivery resulting in a C/S
- STAT C/S

CLINICAL PRESENTATION OF A UTERINE RUPTURE
- Fetal distress
- Stabbing pain at previous C/S incision site
- Vaginal bleeding
- Fetal parts can be easily felt through abdominal wall
- Loss of station
- Unstable maternal VS
- Anticipate a STAT C/S

SOURCES

American College of Obstetricians and Gynecologists. (2004). Vaginal birth after previous cesarean delivery (Practice bulletin no. 54) In *2008 compendium of selected publications* (pp. 825–834). Washington, DC: Author.

Maternity Center. (2009, May 13). *Maternity Center vaginal birth after cesarean.* Unpublished Procedure Manual, Overlook Hospital Department of Ob/Gyn.

VAGINAL DELIVERY

WHAT YOU NEED IN THE ROOM
- Delivery table (should be set if patient is 8 cm or more and should be replaced if not used within 12 hours)
  - Most important instruments are as follows:
    - Scissors
    - Two clamps
  - Bulb suction
- Light source
- lidocaine (Xylocaine)
- oxytocin (Pitocin)
- Sutures
- Syringes (for lidocaine or if emergency drugs need to be administered)
- Step stool
- Cord collection kit if patient is collecting
- Mirror for mother if she wants to see the birth
- Neonatal warmer on
- Neonatal wall suction on to 100 mmHg
- Neonatal O$_2$ on 5 to 10 L/min
- Access to the mother's antenatal blood work
- Blankets
- Oxygen
- Suction
- Diaper
- Infant hat
- Laryngoscope
- Umbilical cord clamp
- Scissors
- Thermometer
- Infant pulsometer
- Erythromycin (erythromycin ophthalmic) ointment 0.5% (*administered in newborn's eyes for prophylaxis against GC/CT*)

■ Vitamin K 1 mg IM × 1 dose (*administered in newborns for prophylaxis of classic hemorrhagic disease*)

WHAT TO DO
■ Monitor FHR
■ Coach mother on pushing
■ Correct ineffective pushing effort
■ Alert other staff that you are in a delivery
■ Note time of birth and delivery of placenta
■ After delivery, place infant on mother's chest (if infant stable)
■ Assess VS
■ Assess Apgar score
■ Place hat on infant
■ Place blanket on infant and mother
■ Encourage breastfeeding
■ If low Apgars
  • Place baby in warmer
  • Notify pediatrician
  • Stimulate baby
■ After delivery of placenta, administer oxytocin (Pitocin) as ordered

HOW TO DO A VAGINAL DELIVERY IN THE ABSENCE OF A PHYSICIAN OR MIDWIFE
■ Apply gloves
■ With one hand apply gentle counter pressure to fetal head
■ With other hand support perineum
■ Once head is out, check for umbilical cord around the neck
■ If loose cord is noted, pull over head
■ If tight cord is noted, use two Kelly clamps and clamp cord
■ Cut between the two clamps

- Allow head to restitute in position
- Apply gentle pressure downward to deliver anterior shoulder
- Apply gentle pressure upward to deliver posterior shoulder
- Slide your posterior hand down the back as the baby delivers, and support feet as they slide over the premium
- If not done already, clamp and cut the cord
- Never pull on the head or use excessive pressure
- Never pull on the umbilical cord while waiting for the placenta

SOURCES

Maternity Center. (2009, May 13). *Maternity Center vaginal delivery.* Unpublished Procedure Manual, Overlook Hospital Department of Ob/Gyn.

Werner, D., Thuman, C., & Manxwell, J. (1992). *Where there is no doctor, a village health care handbook* (Rev. ed.). Berkeley, CA: The Hesperian Foundation.

II

Procedures

As a labor and delivery (L&D) nurse, you will be expected to set up for and assist with various procedures throughout a shift. Because of the nature of this ever-changing unit, any routine procedures can become an emergency very quickly. For this reason, the L&D RN must learn to anticipate possible complications and be prepared to assist both the patient and the physician or midwife.

In this section, you will find information on procedures commonly performed on L&D. The definition, indications, expected outcomes, and complications for each procedure are presented. Keep in mind that this book serves as a general guide to these procedures and does not take the place of practitioner orders or institutional protocol and guidelines. When in doubt, always ask senior nursing staff.

MEDICATIONS TO KNOW
- carboprost (Hemabate)
- methylergonovine (Methergine)
- Rh$_{o}$(D) immunoglobulin, human (IGIM) (RhoGAM)

ABBREVIATIONS TO LEARN
- BPP—biophysical profile
- CPD—cephalopelvic disproportion
- d/t—due to
- fFN—fetal fibronectin
- FHR—fetal heart rate
- HTN—hypertension
- ISE—internal scalp electrode
- IUPC—intrauterine pressure catheter
- NST—nonstress test

EQUIPMENT TO LOCATE AND BECOME FAMILIAR WITH
- Amnihook or Allis clamp
- Electronic fetal monitor (EFM)
- Fetal scalp blood sampling kit
- IUPC catheter
- Proper cable for IUPC
- Types and use of forceps:
  - Simpson's forceps
  - Elliot forceps
  - Kielland forceps
  - Wrigley's forceps
  - Piper's forceps
- Ultrasound (U/S)
- Vacuum (for vacuum delivery)

AMNIOTOMY

Artificial rupture of membranes (ROM) is performed by physician or midwife to induce or expedite labor. May also be done if FHR cannot be obtained through external monitor or if FHR is nonreassuring and placement of ISE and/or IUPC is indicated.

CONTRAINDICATIONS
■ Maternal infection
■ Fetus not engaged in pelvis
■ Placenta previa
■ Presenting part other than head
■ Brow or face presentation

ADVERSE OUTCOMES
■ Cord prolapse
■ Fetal injury
■ Commitment to labor if patient was not in active phase

WHAT YOU NEED
■ Document FHR and fluid color before, during, and after procedure
■ Amnihook or Allis clamp (*should not be used in the presence of polyhydramnios*)
  • For polyhydramnios, offer ISE for puncture of amniotic fluid. *This will allow for a trickle of amniotic fluid instead of a gush that can lead to cord prolapse*
■ Sterile gloves: in appropriate sizes for the physician or midwife
■ Clean white chucks or white towel to place under patient after rupture
■ Assess and document nature of fluid on white chucks or towel to determine if there is meconium

■ Expect continuous leaking of fluid until delivery and gushes with contractions or when patient moves. If FHR changes with decelerations (decels), notify physician or midwife immediately

FAST FACTS in a NUTSHELL

If patient is preterm, discuss with senior or charge nurse before assisting with procedure.

SOURCES

Joseph Hurt, K., Guile, M. W., Bienstock, J. L., Fox, H. E., & Wallach, E. E. (2011). *The Johns Hopkins manual of gynecology and obstetrics* (4th ed.). New York, NY: Lippincott Williams & Wilkins.

Simpson, K. R., & Creehan, P. A. (2008). *Perinatal nursing* (3rd ed.). New York, NY: Lippincott Williams & Wilkins.

AMNIOINFUSION

The process of adding fluid into the uterus through intrauterine catheter. To be done only by a physician or midwife.

INDICATIONS
- Variable decelerations
- Oligohydramnios

CONTRAINDICATIONS
- Malpresentation
- Maternal infection
- Vaginal bleeding of unknown origin
- Placenta previa
- Placental abruption
- Ominous fetal heart tracing
- Umbilical cord prolapse

WHAT YOU NEED
- Sterile gloves
- IUPC catheter (if not already placed)
- IV pump and tubing
- Proper cable for IUPC
- IV fluid (normal saline)

ON PUMP
- Bolus 500 ml of fluid over 30 minutes
- Continuous drip of 100 to 250 ml/hour
- *Bolus and continuous rates should be followed as ordered; if in doubt of proper institutional rates, check policy and procedure manual.*

===============================*FAST FACTS in a NUTSHELL*

Always check to be sure that there is an adequate amount of fluid outflow. If no fluid outflow is noted, notify practitioner immediately and stop infusion.

Guidelines for amniotomy should be followed if membranes are intact before procedure.

SOURCES

Cunningham, G., Leveno, K. J., Bloom, S. L., Hauth, J., Rouse, D., & Spong, C. (2010). *Williams obstetrics* (23rd ed). New York, NY: McGraw-Hill.

Simpson, K. R., & Creehan, P. A. (2008). *Perinatal nursing* (3rd ed.). New York, NY: Lippincott Williams & Wilkins.

Varney, H., Kriebs, J. M., & Gegor, C. L. (2004). *Varney's midwifery* (4th ed.). Sudbury, MA: Jones and Bartlett.

BIOPHYSICAL PROFILE (BPP)

U/S surveillance used to assess the fetal breathing, movements, tone (all must be observed within 30 minutes of each other), and amniotic fluid volume. A nonstress test may not be ordered if U/S assessment is completely normal. To score, each test is rated as 2 (normal) or as 0 (abnormal).

INTERPRETATION OF SCORING
- 8 to 10—reassuring
- 6—equivocal test; should be repeated in 24 hours if patient has not delivered or been induced
- 4 or less—abnormal; patient most likely will be admitted and delivered.

Clinical management will depend on gestational age and full clinical picture.

INDICATIONS
- Postdates
- Intrauterine growth restriction (IUGR)
- Gestational diabetes/type 1 diabetes
- Multiple gestations
- Chronic or pregnancy-induced hypertension
- Hx of fetal demise
- Decreased fetal movement
- Oligohydramnios
- High-risk pregnancy d/t maternal health conditions
- Patient may be assessed as often as 2x/week beginning at 32 weeks; clinical context will predict when to initiate BPP and the frequency.

SOURCES

American College of Obstetricians and Gynecologists. (1999). Antepartum fetal surveillance (Practice bulletin no. 9). In *2008 compendium of selected publications* (pp. 594–595). Washington, DC: Author.

Hurt, J. K., Guile, M. W., Bienstock, J. L., Fox, H. E., & Wallach, E. E. (2011). *The Johns Hopkins manual of gynecology and obstetrics* (4th ed.). New York, NY: Lippincott Williams & Wilkins.

Oyelese, Y., & Vintzileos, A. M. (2011). The uses and limitations of the fetal biophysical profile. *Clinics in Perinatology, 38*(1), 47–64, v–vi.

Varney, H., Kriebs, J. M., & Gegor, C. L. (2004). *Varney's midwifery* (4th ed.). Sudbury, MA: Jones and Bartlett.

EXTERNAL CEPHALIC VERSION

The process in which a breech or transverse fetus is turned into the cephalic position through the abdominal wall. Should only be performed on patients who are 36 weeks of gestation or more.

CONTRAINDICATIONS
- Fetal distress
- Low amniotic fluid
- Placenta previa
- Fetal anomalies
- HTN (uncontrolled or pregnancy induced)
- Uterine malformation

RISKS
- Fetal distress/demise
- Uterine rupture
- Placental abruption
- Labor
- Amniotic fluid embolism
- STAT C/S

WHAT YOU NEED
- First obtain a reactive NST, well documented
- Establish IV access
- Type and screen, complete blood count (CBC)
- If patient is Rh neg, give and document that patient has received RhoGAM
- Blood bank with 2 U on standby
- U/S machine in room
- Gel for mother's abdomen

ORDERS TO BE EXPECTED

■ IV fluids
■ Tocolytics
■ Pain management for mother
■ RhoGAM 300 mcg IM in Rh-neg women after procedure
■ NST after procedure

═══════════════════════════════════*FAST FACTS in a NUTSHELL*

Procedure should ONLY be done if there is an OR with personnel on standby if the need for a STAT C/S occurs.

SOURCES

American College of Obstetricians and Gynecologists. (2000, reaffirmed 2009). *External cephalic version* (Practice bulletin no. 13). Washington, DC: Author, 95(2), 1–7.

Cunningham, G., Leveno, K. J., Bloom, S. L., Hauth, J., Rouse, D., & Spong, C. (2010). *Williams obstetrics* (23rd ed.). New York, NY: McGraw-Hill.

FETAL FIBRONECTIN (fFN)

Vaginal swab that is used to predict the likelihood a patient will go into labor within the next 2 weeks. Should be done between 24 and 34 weeks and every 2 weeks as indicated.

INDICATIONS
- History of preterm delivery
- Symptoms of preterm labor

WHAT YOU NEED
- Speculum
- Sterile gloves
- Adequate light source
- fFN swab

TEST WILL BE INACCURATE IF
- ROM
- Bleeding present
- Patient has had sex or vaginal exam within 24 hours of the test
- Medication or lubrication present
- Cervix is dilated greater than 3 cm
- Patient has vaginal infection

INTERPRETATION OF RESULTS
- Negative = 99% that patient will not deliver within 7 to 10 days
- Positive = 87% that patient will deliver within 7 days

SOURCES

fFNTest.com. (2011). *fFNTest online*. Retrieved from www.ffntest
.com/hcp/testing/specimen_collection.html

Hurt, K. J., Guile, M. W., Bienstock, J. L., Fox, H. E., & Wallach, E. E.
(2011). *The Johns Hopkins manual of gynecology and obstetrics*
(4th ed.). New York, NY: Lippincott Williams & Wilkins.

Lab Tests Online. (2011). *Lab Tests Online*. Retrieved from www
.labtestsonline.org/understanding/analytes/ffn/tab/test

FETAL SCALP SAMPLING

Obtaining blood from the scalp of the fetus to determine if there is adequate oxygenation to the fetus.

INDICATIONS
- Equivocal FHR without imminent delivery

CONTRAINDICATIONS
- Mother is HIV or hepatitis positive
- Cervical dilatation less than 3 cm
- Present part other than head
- Membranes must be ruptured

WHAT YOU NEED
- Fetal scalp blood sampling kit:
  - Endoscopic tube
  - Heparinized capillary tubes
  - Blood gas analyzer
- Adequate light
- Long 2-mm blade if not in kit
- Betadine for cleansing head

INTERPRETING RESULTS

Interpretation	pH	Action
Normal	>7.25	Repeat test in 20–30 min
Preacidotic	7.20–7.24	Repeat test in 5 min
Fetal acidosis	<7.20	Two collections 5 min apart; prepare for immediate delivery

WHAT TO DO

If a midwife is managing this patient, notify the backup physician if fetal heart tones (FHT) warrant this test to be performed.

SOURCES

Hurt, K. J., Guile, M. W., Bienstock, J. L., Fox, H. E., & Wallach, E. E. (2011). *The Johns Hopkins manual of gynecology and obstetrics* (4th ed.). New York, NY: Lippincott Williams & Wilkins.

Simpson, K. R., & Creehan, P. A. (2008). *Perinatal nursing* (3rd ed.). New York, NY: Lippincott Williams & Wilkins.

Varney, H., Kriebs, J. M., & Gegor, C. L. (2004). *Varney's midwifery* (4th ed.). Sudbury, MA: Jones and Bartlett.

NONSTRESS TEST (NST)

Evaluation of fetal well-being using EFM to monitor FHR.

INDICATIONS
- Decreased fetal movement
- Postdates
- Maternal history of gestational diabetes mellitus (GDM) or DM type I or II
- Maternal HTN
- Known fetal anomalies
- IUGR
- Twins
- Abnormal amniotic fluid index
- Poor maternal weight gain
- Maternal history of intrauterine fetal demise (IUFD)

WHAT YOU NEED
- Toco
- EFM
- Gel for monitor
- Bands to keep monitor in place

REACTIVE NST
- Fetal heart baseline should be between 110 and 160
- Less than 32 weeks, two or more accelerations rising 10 bpm above baseline for 10 seconds each
- Greater than 32 weeks, two or more accelerations rising 15 bpm above baseline for 15 seconds each

NONREACTIVE NST
Failure to meet above criteria within a 40-minute time frame.

SOURCES

American College of Obstetricians and Gynecologists. (1999). Antepartum fetal surveillance (Practice bulletin no. 9). In *2008 compendium of selected publications* (pp. 592–602). Washington, DC: Author.

Maternity Center. (2010, June 6). *Maternity Center: Non-stress testing.* Unpublished Procedure Manual, Overlook Hospital Department of Ob/Gyn.

OPERATIVE VAGINAL DELIVERY

The use of either forceps or vacuum to assist with a vaginal delivery.

INDICATIONS
- Maternal exhaustion
- Inadequate/prolonged pushing
- Fetal distress
- Cardiac delivery

COMPLICATIONS
- Maternal lacerations: cervical, vaginal, and possible damage to anal sphincter
- Episiotomy
- Postpartum hemorrhage
- Trauma to urethra and/or bladder
- Newborn lacerations
- Skull fracture
- Nerve damage: maternal and fetal
- Intracranial bleed

REQUIREMENTS
- Fully dilated
- Fetal head engaged in pelvis
- Maternal bladder empty
- No suspicion of CPD
- Gestation age greater than 36 weeks

WHAT TO DO
- Notify pediatrician
- Set up room for vaginal delivery
- Place forceps or vacuum on delivery table in a sterile manner

- Have methylergonovine (Methergine) and carboprost (Hemabate) available
- Place stepping stool in room
- Request a more senior nurse to assist with delivery

TYPES OF FORCEPS
- Simpson's forceps: most common
- Elliot forceps: should only be used in multiparous women
- Kielland forceps: used for rotating the baby
- Wrigley's forceps: used in low or outlet delivery
- Piper's forceps: used in breech deliveries

CRITERIA OF FORCEPS
- Outlet forceps: fetal scalp remains visible when mother is not pushing
- Low forceps: fetal station is +2 or below
- Midforceps: fetal head engaged but above +2 station

VACUUM DELIVERY
- General rule maximum of three pulls
- Popoffs indicate too much force without progression of fetal head descent
  - They should not be accepted as routine and a maximum of three popoffs should indicate need for other methods of delivery
- No more than 600 mmHg of pressure should be used
- Maximum vacuum time from placement until detachment or delivery should not exceed 30 minutes

SOURCES

Cunningham, G., Leveno, K. J., Bloom, S. L., Hauth, J., Rouse, D., & Spong, C. (2010). *Williams obstetrics* (23rd ed.). New York, NY: McGraw-Hill.

Healthline. (2011). *Healthline online.* Retrieved from www.healthline .com/yodocontent/pregnancy/assisted-delivery-types-forceps .html

Maternity Center. (2007, May 23). *Maternity Center vacuum extractor.* Unpublished Procedure Manual, Overlook Hospital Department of Ob/Gyn.

Simpson, K. R., & Creehan, P. A. (2008). *Perinatal nursing* (3rd ed.). New York, NY: Lippincott Williams & Wilkins.

PART

III

Emergencies

As labor and delivery (L&D) is a fast-paced unit, many hospitals consider it an ICU and limit the number of patients assigned per RN to two. This is because complications can (and do) arise without notice. On "good days," the majority of your patients will be healthy with a normal progression of labor, and delivery of a healthy beautiful newborn. On "other days," your patients might be acutely ill with complications related or unrelated to the pregnancy.

These are the patients whom you must observe carefully for subtle changes in either the mother or the baby, and know how to respond immediately when necessary to those changes. You are the first line of care for your patient. It is your responsibility to be informed of potential complications and, when related changes occur, to tell the physician or midwife of these changes immediately.

In this section, you will find the more common complications and emergencies that you will encounter in L&D. This is an important section. Read it over and over until you feel totally familiar with the content so that you can act competently and appropriately when a complication arises. During an actual emergency, there is little time to refer to a reference book.

MEDICATIONS TO KNOW
- ampicillin
- gentamicin
- clindamycin (Cleocin)
- erythromycin (Erythrocin)
- vancomycin (Vancocin)
- magnesium sulfate
- calcium gluconate
- labetalol (Trandate)
- hydralazine
- betamethasone (Celestone)
- dexamethasone
- lorazepam (Ativan)
- oxytocin (Pitocin)
- methylergonovine (Methergine)
- carboprost (Hemabate)
- misoprostol (Cytotec)
- indomethacin (Indocin)
- nifedipine (Procardia)
- terbutaline
- dinoprostone (Cervidil, Prepidil)

ABBREVIATIONS TO LEARN
- C/S—cesarean section
- DIC—disseminated intracoagulopathy
- HELLP—hemolysis elevated liver enzymes low platelet count
- PPH—postpartum hemorrhage
- PPROM—preterm premature rupture of membranes
- U/S—ultrasound

EQUIPMENT TO LOCATE AND TO BECOME FAMILIAR WITH
- Neonate crash cart

ABRUPTIO PLACENTAE

Separation of placenta from uterine wall before delivery.

RISK FACTORS
- Scar on uterus (prior myomectomy or C/S)
- Blunt abdominal trauma
- Hx of previous abruptio placentae
- Hypertension (HTN)
- Multiparity
- PPROM
- Cocaine use
- AMA
- Smoking

CLINICAL PRESENTATION
- Acute localized uterine pain
- Frank bleeding
- Occult bleeding (need U/S to determine)
- Back pain
- Fetal distress

WHOM TO CALL
- GET HELP IMMEDIATELY
- Physician/midwife to bedside immediately
- Senior nursing staff
- Alert on-call pediatrician
- Rapid response team/code team

WHAT TO DO
- Establish continuous fetal heart rate (FHR)
- Anticipate possible need for internal fetal monitoring
- IV access with 18G needle (if not already done)
- Monitor maternal vital signs (VS)

- Call blood bank and have 2 U of packed RBC cross matched
- Anticipate probable C/S (not always indicated)
- Obtain portable U/S in room

LABS

- Complete blood count (CBC)
- Type and screen
- PT/PTT
- Fibrinogen
- Fibrin split products
- Toxicology

FAST FACTS in a NUTSHELL

- *Patients with abruption may have precipitous deliveries*
- *Anticipate possible PPH or DIC.*

SOURCES

Cunningham, G., Leveno, K. J., Bloom, S. L., Hauth, J., Rouse, D., & Spong, C. (2010). *Williams obstetrics* (23rd ed.). New York, NY: McGraw-Hill.

Joseph Hurt, K., Guile, M. W., Bienstock, J. L., Fox, H. E., & Wallach, E. E. (2011). *The Johns Hopkins manual of gynecology and obstetrics* (4th ed.). New York, NY: Lippincott Williams & Wilkins.

Pariente, G., Wiznitzer, A., Sergienko, R., Mazor, M., Holcberg, G., & Sheiner, E. (2011). Placental abruption: Critical analysis of risk factors and perinatal outcomes. *Journal of Maternal-Fetal & Neonatal Medicine, 24*(5), 698–702.

Simpson, K. R., & Creehan, P. A. (2008). *Perinatal nursing* (3rd ed.). New York, NY: Lippincott Williams & Wilkins.

AMNIOTIC FLUID EMBOLISM

It is a rare complication where amniotic fluid or fetal debris crosses the placenta into maternal circulation. It can occur during labor or postpartum.

RISK FACTORS
- Induction of labor
- Operative delivery
- Mutiparity
- Advanced maternal age
- Placenta previa
- Abdominal trauma

CLINICAL PRESENTATION
- Dyspnea
- Cyanosis
- Fetal distress (if undelivered)
- Maternal hypotension
- Maternal cardiac arrest

WHOM TO CALL
- GET HELP IMMEDIATELY
- Call covering physician STAT if midwife is managing patient
- Anesthesia STAT
- All senior nursing staff available to help

WHAT TO DO
- Give O_2 through facemask
- Call blood bank for
  - Two units of packed RBC crossed and matched brought STAT
  - Fresh frozen plasma STAT

- Access another IV site with 18G needle
- Anticipate STAT C/S and full maternal code (prep patient for C/S and have crash cart ready)

LABS
- Type and screen (if admission labs not obtained)
- Arterial blood gases
- Serum electrolytes
- CMP
- Coagulation profile
- CBC

FAST FACTS in a NUTSHELL

If patient survives delivery, high risk for DIC.

SOURCES

Cunningham, G., Leveno, K. J., Bloom, S. L., Hauth, J., Rouse, D., & Spong, C. (2010). *Williams obstetrics* (23rd ed.). New York, NY: McGraw-Hill.

Curran, C. A. (2003). Intrapartum emergencies. *Journal of Obstetric, Gynecologic, & Neonatal Nursing, 32*, 802–813. doi:10.1177/0884217503258425

Hurt, K. J., Guile, M. W., Bienstock, J. L., Fox, H. E., & Wallach, E. E. (2011). *The Johns Hopkins manual of gynecology and obstetrics* (4th ed.). New York, NY: Lippincott Williams & Wilkins.

BLEEDING IN PREGNANCY

Causes in second and third trimester

Painful	Painless
Labor term or preterm	Placenta previa
Placenta abruption	Loss of mucus plug
Uterine rupture	Polyp on cervix (mostly seen after intercourse)
Trauma	

=======*FAST FACTS in a NUTSHELL*

Never do a vaginal exam if cause of bleeding is unknown. Notify practitioner immediately.

WHAT TO DO
- Call practitioner on call
- Call senior nursing staff
- Maternal VS
- Monitor fetus with electronic fetal monitoring (EFM) and Toco
- Start IV fluids LR

WHAT YOU WILL NEED
- Bedpan (if patient is in a triage stretcher of a bed that does not break)
  - For examination, place bedpan upside down under the patient's buttocks
- Sterile gloves
- Sterile speculum
- Proper lighting

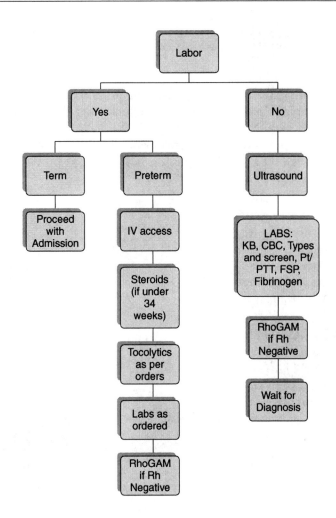

SOURCES

Cunningham, G., Leveno, K. J., Bloom, S. L., Hauth, J., Rouse, D., & Spong, C. (2010). *Williams obstetrics* (23rd ed.). New York, NY: McGraw-Hill.

Hurt, K. J., Guile, M. W., Bienstock, J. L., Fox, H. E., & Wallach, E. E. (2011). *The Johns Hopkins manual of gynecology and obstetrics* (4th ed.). New York, NY: Lippincott Williams & Wilkins.

BREECH

TYPES
- Footling: (incomplete) extension of one or both hips
- Complete: presenting part is buttocks and flexion is noted in both knees and hips
- Frank: presenting part is buttocks and there is extension through the knees (feet are near head)

RISK FACTORS
- Multiple gestations
- Bicornuate uterus
- Fibroids
- Preterm labor
- Polyhydramnios
- Macrosomia

ADVERSE EFFECTS
- Cord prolapse
- Fetal injury
- Fetal asphyxia
- Mortality
- Head entrapment (cervix may not be fully dilated)

WHAT TO DO
- Delivery eminent
  - CALL FOR HELP, NOTIFY PEDIATRICIAN STAT
  - Monitor fetus
  - If cord prolapse noted, put mother in Trendelenburg and try to relieve pressure on umbilical cord using a vaginal hand (see umbilical cord prolapse)
- Delivery not eminent
  - Monitor fetus
  - Call the on-call practitioner STAT
  - Prep for C/S

WHAT YOU NEED FOR A VAGINAL BREECH DELIVERY

- Delivery tray (at least a pair of sterile scissors and lidocaine)
- For leverage bring the mother to edge of bed or break the bed, if time
- Warm towel (practitioner will need during delivery to apply around neonate's body)
- IV access: 18G needle
- Neonate crash cart
- Pediatrician in room

SOURCES

Cunningham, G., Leveno, K. J., Bloom, S. L., Hauth, J., Rouse, D., & Spong, C. (2010). *Williams obstetrics* (23rd ed.). New York, NY: McGraw-Hill.

Hurt, K. J., Guile, M. W., Bienstock, J. L., Fox, H. E., & Wallach, E. E. (2011). *The Johns Hopkins manual of gynecology and obstetrics* (4th ed.). New York, NY: Lippincott Williams & Wilkins.

Varney, H., Kriebs, J. M., & Gegor, C. L. (2004). *Varney's midwifery* (4th ed.). Sudbury, MA: Jones and Bartlett.

CHORIOAMNIONITIS

Infection of placenta, chorion, and amnion.

RISK FACTORS
- Prolonged labor
- PROM/PPROM
- Serial vaginal exams
- Intrauterine pressure catheter (IUPC)/internal scalp electrode (ISE)
- Vaginal infections (i.e., bacterial vaginosis [BV] or group B streptococcus [GBS])

CLINICAL PRESENTATION

Maternal	Fetal
Temp of 38° C	Tachycardia
Tachycardia	Amniotic fluid has foul odor
Increased WBC	Low Apgars
Tender abdomen	Acidosis
Labor dystocia	

WHAT TO EXPECT
- Induction of labor
- Augmentation to hasten labor
- VS ordered q hour
- Antibiotic therapy (note whether the patient has allergies)
- After vaginal delivery, antibiotics usually discontinued
- Antibiotics to be administered will continue for 24 to 48 hours after last maternal temp

- No PCN allergy
- ampicillin 2 g intravenous piggyback (IVPB) × 1 dose, then 1 g 4 hr
- gentamicin 120 mg IVPB × 1 dose, then 80 mg IVPB q 8 hr
- PCN allergy
- clindamycin (Cleocin) 900 mg IVPB q 8 hr
- erythromycin (Erythrocin) 1 g IVPB q 6 hr
- vancomycin (Vancocin) 500 mg IVPB q 6 hr

FAST FACTS in a NUTSHELL

Pediatrician should be notified and present at the delivery.

SOURCES

American College of Obstetricians and Gynecologists. (2003). Dystocia and augmentation of labor (Practice bulletin no. 49). In *2008 compendium of selected publications* (p. 804). Washington, DC: Author.

Hurt, K. J., Guile, M. W., Bienstock, J. L., Fox, H. E., & Wallach, E. E. (2011). *The Johns Hopkins manual of gynecology and obstetrics* (4th ed.). New York, NY: Lippincott Williams & Wilkins.

Varney, H., Kriebs, J. M., & Gegor, C. L. (2004). *Varney's midwifery* (4th ed.). Sudbury, MA: Jones and Bartlett.

HYPERTENSION IN PREGNANCY

PREECLAMPSIA

Develops after 20 weeks' gestation and patient is usually symptomatic with proteinuria, HA, visual disturbances, and epigastric pain. Cause is unknown.

DIAGNOSIS
- 140 systolic or 90 diastolic or higher after 20 weeks' gestational diabetes (GA) with no hx of HTN
- Proteinuria >0.3 g/d in 24-hour urine
- *Severe preeclampsia*
- 160 mmHg systolic and 110 mmHg diastolic
- Proteinuria 5 g or more in results of 24-hour urine collection
- Oliguria less than 500 ml in 24-hour urine results

RISK FACTORS
- Primip
- Multiple gestations
- Diabetes
- Teen pregnancy
- AMA

COMPLICATIONS
- Seizure
- HELLP syndrome
- Intrauterine growth restriction (IUGR)
- Abruptio placentae

LABS
- CBC
- Liver function panel
- Kidney function panel

- PT/PTT
- Fibrinogen
- Urine dipstick/urinalysis
- 24-hour urine collection

LAB INTERPRETATION
- Elevated
  - LDH
  - Serum creatinine
  - Uric acid >6 mg
  - AST/ALT
  - Proteinuria

MEDICATIONS (ADMINISTER AS ORDERED)
Seizure Prevention
- Magnesium sulfate loading dose 4 to 6 g IV then 2 to 4 g IV/hr
  - Serum Mg level should be drawn q 6 hr. Levels should be between 6 and 8 mg/dl
    - Mg levels 8 to 10 mg/dl decrease deep tendon reflexes
      - 13 to 15 mg/dl respiratory distress
      - >15 mg/dl cardiac arrest
  - Monitor I&Os and IV fluid needs to be managed, so no more than 125 ml/hour of total if IV fluids is infusing
  - ANTIDOTE (hypermagnesemia): Calcium gluconate 1 g IV over 3 min
    - Should be in room if $MgSO_4$ is infusing

HTN Control
- labetalol (Trandate) 20 mg IV push, then escalating 10-minute intervals of 20, 40, 80 mg for max 300 mg/24 hr
  - Not for RN administration
- Hydralazine 5 mg IV bolus q 20 min until 20 mg PRN

Steroids for Fetal Lung Maturity If Preterm
- betamethasone (Celestone) 12 mg IM q 24 hr × 2
- dexamethasone 6 mg IM q 12 hr × 4

HELLP SYNDROME

Acronym stands for, H—hemolysis, EL—elevated liver enzymes, LP—low platelet count
   Risk factors, symptoms, and treatment similar to preeclampsia

LABS
- CBC
- Liver function panel
- Kidney function panel
- PT/PTT
- Fibrinogen
- Urine dipstick/urinalysis
- 24-hour urine collection

LAB INTERPRETATION
- Hemolysis
- Increased liver enzymes
- Low platelets

ECLAMPSIA

Preceded by preeclampsia, but patient has suffered from seizure activity and/or coma

MANAGEMENT OF A SEIZURE
Whom to Call
- GET HELP IMMEDIATELY
- Notify attending physician STAT

- Notify anesthesia STAT
- All senior nursing staff available to help
- Notify pediatrician: should be on standby for STAT C/S

What to Do

- Secure the area so that the patient is safe while having seizure
- ABCs
- Give O_2 through facemask
- Anticipate fetal bradycardia
- Access another IV site with 18G needle
- Anticipate STAT C/S once FHR has stabilized or has been bradycardic for longer than 10 minutes

Medications (administer as ordered)

- Magnesium sulfate 6 g IV bolus
  - If seizure occurs during or after loading dose, bolus another 2 g

If seizure activity persists,

lorazepam (Ativan) 0.1 mg/kg IV (most likely administered by anesthesia)

SOURCES

American College of Obstetricians and Gynecologists. (2001). Chronic hypertension in pregnancy (Practice bulletin no. 29). In *2008 compendium of selected publications* (pp. 686–694). Washington, DC: Author.

American College of Obstetricians and Gynecologists. (2002). Diagnosis and management of preeclampsia and eclampsia (Practice bulletin no. 33). In *2008 compendium of selected publications* (pp. 717–725). Washington, DC: Author.

Hurt, K. J., Guile, M. W., Bienstock, J. L., Fox, H. E., & Wallach, E. E. (2011). *The Johns Hopkins manual of gynecology and obstetrics* (4th ed.). New York, NY: Lippincott Williams & Wilkins.

NEONATAL RESUSCITATION

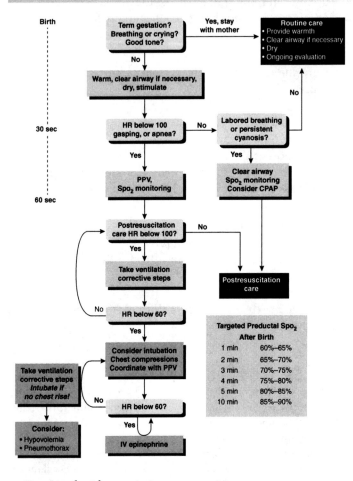

Reprinted with permission.

SOURCE

American Heart Association. (2011). *Newborn resuscitation algo-rithm.* Retrieved from http://circ.ahajournals.org/content/122/18_suppl_3/S909/F1.expansion.html

PLACENTAL ABNORMALITIES

PLACENTA PREVIA

As the uterus grows, the placenta moves and previas may resolve by time of delivery. U/S is needed to rule out previous previa at term if not already done.

DEFINITIONS
- Low lying: the placenta is close to the edge of os
- Marginal: the placenta has reached the edge of the os
- Partial: the placenta is covering some of the os
- Complete: the placenta is completely covering the os
- Vasa previa: cord insertion is through membranes instead of placenta

RISK FACTORS
- Multiparity
- Prior uterine surgery
- AMA
- Smoking
- Abnormality of uterus

═══════════════════════════════════FAST FACTS in a NUTSHELL

Sterile vaginal exam (SVE) and vaginal delivery are contraindicated.

If patient with known previa presents with painless vaginal bleeding

WHOM TO CALL
- GET HELP IMMEDIATELY
- Call covering physician STAT if midwife is managing patient
- Notify anesthesia STAT
- Notify pediatrician STAT
- Call all senior nursing staff available to help

WHAT TO DO
- DO NOT DO A VAGINAL EXAM
- Prepare for a STAT C/S
  - Start IV LR 18G
  - Admission labs
  - Blood bank 2 U crossed and matched
  - Bicitra (if time)
  - Foley catheter
  - Consent
  - ID bands
- Monitor FHR

PLACENTA ACCRETA/INCRETA/ PERCRETA

May be diagnosed after delivery of neonate when the placenta fails to deliver as expected. Patient may be taken to OR for postdelivery dilatation and curettage (D&C) or possible hysterectomy if bleeding cannot be controlled.

DEFINITIONS
- Accreta: placenta attaches to myometrium without the decidua basalis
- Increta: attaches into the myometrium
- Percreta: placenta permeates through the myometrium and may affect the bladder and/or bowel

WHAT TO EXPECT
▧ Possible C/S hysterectomy

SOURCES

Cunningham, G., Leveno, K. J., Bloom, S. L., Hauth, J., Rouse, D., & Spong, C. (2010). *Williams obstetrics* (23rd ed.). New York, NY: McGraw-Hill.

Hurt, K. J., Guile, M. W., Bienstock, J. L., Fox, H. E., & Wallach, E. E. (2011). *The Johns Hopkins manual of gynecology and obstetrics* (4th ed.). New York, NY: Lippincott Williams & Wilkins.

Simpson, K. R., & Creehan, P. A. (2008). *Perinatal nursing* (3rd ed.). New York, NY: Lippincott Williams & Wilkins.

POSTPARTUM HEMORRHAGE

Greater than 1,000 ml of blood loss after vaginal or cesarean delivery. Hemodynamic instability may occur with less blood loss if patient is anemic. Can also be diagnosed with a 10% drop of hematocrit (HCT).

RISK FACTORS
- Anemia
- Overdistended uterus
- Pitocin induction/augmentation
- Infection
- Retained placenta
- Prolonged labor
- Fibroids
- Lacerations during delivery
- Operative delivery
- Maternal coagulation deficiencies

WHAT TO DO
- GET HELP IMMEDIATELY
- Start IV 18G (if not previously done)
- Empty bladder with catheter
- Monitor maternal VS
- Give O_2 through nonrebreather facemask
- Administration of Methergine/Hemabate/Pitocin as ordered
- Call blood bank: 2 U crossed and matched STAT
- Anticipate possible transfer to OR for D&C or hysterectomy if bleeding is unable to be controlled

MEDICATIONS (ADMINISTER AS ORDERED)
- oxytocin (Pitocin): 10 IU/ml IM or 40 U IV—should have in room at every delivery
- methylergonovine (Methergine): 0.2 mg IM q 2 to 4 hr—do not give to HTN/preeclamptic patients
  - SHOULD BE KEPT IN REFRIGERATOR

- carboprost (Hemabate) 250 mcg IM q 15 to 90 min max eight doses
- Do not give with hx of asthma
- misoprostol (Cytotec) 800 to 1,000 mcg rectal
- dinoprostone (Cervidil, Prepidil) 20 mg PR/PV q 2 hr

SOURCES

American College of Obstetricians and Gynecologists. (2006). Postpartum hemorrhage (Practice bulletin no. 76). In *2008 compendium of selected publications* (pp. 911–917). Washington, DC: Author.

Varney, H., Kriebs, J. M., & Gegor, C. L. (2004). *Varney's midwifery* (4th ed.). Sudbury, MA: Jones and Bartlett.

PREMATURITY

PRETERM L&D

Between the weeks of 20 and 37 gestational age with regular uterine contractions (UCX) and cervical dilatation or rupture of membranes (ROM)

RISK FACTORS
- Multiple gestations
- Infection
- No prenatal care
- Smoking
- Substance abuse

WHAT TO DO
- Monitor FHR and UCX patterns
- Start IV and hydrate
- Maternal VS
- Admission labs
- Evaluation of PROM
- Anticipate sterile speculum exam

WHAT TO EXPECT
- Anticipate sterile speculum exam
- Fetal fibronectin (fFN)
- Admission
- Anticipate delivery if above 34 weeks and PPROM

LABS
- CBC
- Urinalysis
- Urine culture and sensitivity (obtained through straight catheter)
- Vaginal cultures

MEDICATIONS (administer as ordered)

■ Corticosteroids—for fetal lung maturity (between 24 and 34 weeks)
  • betamethasone (Celestone) 12 mg IM q 12 hr × 2 doses
  • Dexamethasone 6 mg IM q 12 hr × 4 doses
■ Tocolytics—to try and stop labor
  • indomethacin (Indocin) 50 to 100 mg PO at first dose, then 25 to 50 mg PO q 4 to 6 hr
    • Do not give if oligohydramnios
  • nifedipine (Procardia) 10 to 20 mg PO q 6 hr
  • Terbutaline 0.25 mg SQ q 20 to 30 min PRN
    • May cause maternal tachycardia
  • Magnesium sulfate loading dose 4 to 6 g IV, then 2 to 4 g IV/hr
    • Serum Mg level should be drawn q 6 hr. Levels should be between 6 and 8 mg/dl
      • Mg levels 8 to 10 mg/dl decrease deep tendon reflexes
        • 13 to 15 mg/dl respiratory distress
        • >15 mg/dl cardiac arrest
  • Monitor I&Os and IV fluid needs to be managed, so that no more than 125 ml/hr of total IV fluids is infusing

═══════════════════════════════════════*FAST FACTS in a NUTSHELL*

ANTIDOTE [hypermagnesemia]: calcium gluconate 1 g IV over 3 minutes; should be in room if MgSO$_4$ is infusing.

■ Antibiotics—If PPROM
  • Ampicillin 2 g IV q 6 hr × 48 hr, then
  • erythromycin (Erythrocin) 250 mg IV q 6 hr × 48 hr

SOURCES

American College of Obstetricians and Gynecologists. (2003). Management of preterm labor (Practice bulletin no. 43). In *2008 compendium of selected publications* (pp. 765–773). Washington, DC: Author.

Hurt, K. J., Guile, M. W., Bienstock, J. L., Fox, H. E., & Wallach, E. E. (2011). *The Johns Hopkins manual of gynecology and obstetrics* (4th ed.). New York, NY: Lippincott Williams & Wilkins.

Varney, H., Kriebs, J. M., & Gegor, C. L. (2004). *Varney's midwifery* (4th ed.). Sudbury, MA: Jones and Bartlett.

SHOULDER DYSTOCIA

- Obstetrical emergency
- The fetus' anterior shoulder is lodged behind the woman's pubic bone.

RISK FACTORS
- Maternal hx of shoulder dystocia with previous deliveries
- Macrosomia
- Gestation diabetes
- Maternal obesity
- Postdates
- Undiagnosed cephalopelvic disproportion (CPD)

CLINICAL PRESENTATION
- Turtle sign is a classic sign of an impending shoulder dystocia. After the head emerges from the vagina it quickly retracts.
- Dysfunctional second stage or active phase of labor (not always seen)

WHOM TO CALL
- GET HELP IMMEDIATELY
- Call covering physician STAT if midwife is managing patient
- Notify pediatrician STAT
- Notify anesthesia STAT
- Call all senior nursing staff available to help

FAST FACTS in a NUTSHELL

ALWAYS HAVE A STEP STOOL IN DELIVERY ROOM.

WHAT TO DO

- ▦ Instruct mother NOT to push until instructed to do so; explain there is a problem and provide reassurance
- ▦ Strategies that may serve to alleviate or dislodge shoulder dystocia
- ▦ McRoberts maneuver: bring mother's legs all the way back in an exaggerated lithotomy position (this will open diameter of the pelvis)

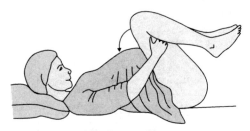

Lithotomy position

- ▦ Apply suprapubic pressure: ask the practitioner which way the back is. Angle pressure diagonally against fetal back in attempt to collapse the anterior shoulder.
  - • DO NOT PRESS STRAIGHT DOWN

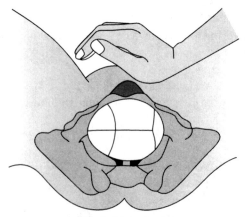

Suprapubic pressure

FAST FACTS in a NUTSHELL

DO NOT APPLY FUNDAL PRESSURE.

- Be prepared to readjust and do McRoberts maneuver again
- Gaskin position: hands and knee position may be requested by the practitioner, assist mother into this position

WHAT THE PHYSICIAN AND/OR MIDWIFE IS DOING

- Although the RN is aiding with the dislodgment of the shoulder externally, the practitioner is attempting to use internal maneuvers to dislodge the shoulders
- Rubin's maneuver: internally trying to collapse anterior shoulder to dislodge from pubic bone

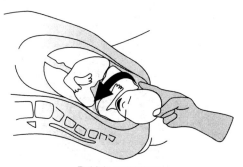

Rubin's maneuver

■ Woods' screw maneuver: rotating the posterior shoulder into anterior position to facilitate delivery of the neonate

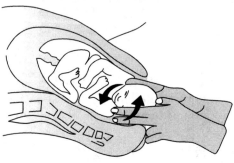

Woods' screw maneuver

■ Reverse Woods' screw maneuver: similar to Woods' screw maneuver but rotating in opposite direction

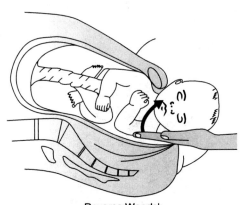

Reverse Woods'
screw maneuver

- Delivery of the posterior arm: sweeping the posterior arm across the fetal chest delivering the position shoulder first

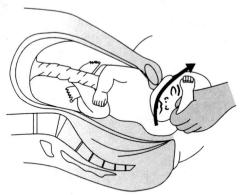

Delivery of the posterior arm

- Zananelli maneuver: if all efforts fail to deliver vaginally, Zananelli maneuver is performed to replace the fetus back into the vaginal canal and proceed with cesarean delivery.

ANTICIPATE

- Full neonate code
- Postpartum hemorrhage

SOURCES

Varney, H., Kriebs, J. M., & Gegor, C. L. (2004). *Varney's midwifery* (4th ed.). Sudbury, MA: Jones and Bartlett.

Medical Illustrations

South Australian Perinatal Practice Guidelines. (2010). *Shoulder dystocia*. Retrieved from www.health.sa.gov.au/PPG/DEFAULT .aspx?PageContentMode=1&tabid=210

UMBILICAL CORD PROLAPSE

Fetal blood supply compromised because the umbilical cord has slipped through the cervix ahead of the presenting part (frank) or has slipped alongside of presenting part (occult). Both are medical emergencies, and a STAT cesarean delivery should be anticipated.

RISK FACTORS
- Preterm
- Polyhydramnios
- Multiple gestations
- ROM before fetal head is engaged in pelvis
- Malpresentation

CLINICAL PRESENTATION
- Usually occurs immediately after ROM
- Prolonged bradycardia
- Severe variable decelerations
- Umbilical cord palpable on vaginal exam
- Visualization of cord inside vagina
- Visualization of cord prolapsing from vagina

WHOM TO CALL
- GET HELP IMMEDIATELY
- Call covering physician STAT if midwife is managing patient
- Notify pediatrician STAT
- Notify anesthesia STAT

WHAT TO DO
- Occult cord: position mother in knee to chest or Trendelenburg position
- Continue to attempt to assess FHR either through EFM, ISE (if previously placed), or U/S

- Frank cord: Place hand in vagina and push presenting part off the cord
  - DO NOT REMOVE HAND FROM VAGINA until instructed to do so by the practitioner during C/S
- Wrap cord in towel soaked with warm normal saline
- Anticipate STAT C/S

SOURCES

Hurt, K. J., Guile, M. W., Bienstock, J. L., Fox, H. E., & Wallach, E. E. (2011). *The Johns Hopkins manual of gynecology and obstetrics* (4th ed.). New York, NY: Lippincott Williams & Wilkins.

Varney, H., Kriebs, J. M., & Gegor, C. L. (2004). *Varney's midwifery* (4th ed.). Sudbury, MA: Jones and Bartlett.

Abbreviations

ACOG	American College of Obstetricians and Gynecologists
AFI/AFV	amniotic fluid index/volume
AFP	alpha fetoprotein
AROM	artificial rupture of membranes
ASCUS	atypical squamous cells of undetermined significance
B-hCG	beta-human chorionic gonadotropin
BID	two times a day
BP	blood pressure
bpm	beats per minute
BPP	biophysical profile
BV	bacterial vaginosis
c/o	complaint of
C/S	cesarean section
C&S	culture and sensitivity
CBC	complete blood count
CC	chief complaint
CF	cystic fibrosis
CIN	cervical intraepithelia neoplasia
CM	certified midwife

CMT	cervical motion tenderness
CMV	cytomegalovirus
CNM	certified nurse midwife
CNS	central nervous system
colpo	colposcopy
complete	10 cm dilated
CP	cerebral palsy
CPD	cephalopelvic disproportion
CT	*Chlamydia trachomatis*
ctx	uterine contractions
CVS	chorionic villa sampling
CXR	chest x-ray
d/c	discontinue
d/t	due to
D&C	dilatation and curettage
DES	diethylstilbestrol
DIC	disseminated intracoagulopathy
DKA	diabetic ketoacidosis
DM	diabetes mellitus
DOB	date of birth
DTR	deep tendon reflex
DVT	deep vein thrombosis
dx	diagnosis
EDC/EDD	estimated date of confinement/delivery date
EFM	electronic fetal monitoring
EFW	estimated fetal weight
F/U	follow-up
fFN	fetal fibronectin
FHR/FHT	fetal heart rate/tones
FKC	fetal kick count
FOB	father of baby

FSE	fetal scalp electrode
g	gram
GA	gestational diabetes
GBS	group B streptococcus
GC	gonorrhea
GCT	glucose challenge test
GDM	gestational diabetes mellitus
GTT	glucose tolerance test
GU	genitourinary
GYN	gynecological
H/A	headache
Hb	hemoglobin
HCT	hematocrit
HDN	hemorrhagic disease of the newborn
HEENT	head, ears, eyes, nose, throat
h/o	history of
HPI	history of present illness
HPV	human papilloma virus
hs	hour of sleep
HSIL	high-grade squamous intraepithelial lesions
HSV	herpes simplex virus
HTN	hypertension
hx	history
IA	intermittent auscultation
IDDM	insulin-dependent diabetes
IM	intramuscular
IP	intrapartum
ISE	internal scalp electrode
ITP	idiopathic thrombocytopenia
IU	international units
IUFD	intrauterine fetal demise

IUGR	intrauterine growth restriction
IUI	intrauterine insemination
IUP	intrauterine pregnancy
IUPC	intrauterine pressure catheter
IV	intravenous
IVF	in vitro fertilization
IVPB	intravenous piggyback
L/S	lecithin/spinogomyelin
LBW	low birth weight
LGA	large for gestational age
LMP	last menstrual period
LSIL	low-grade squamous intraepithelial lesions
mcg	microgram
mg	milligram
ml	milliliter
MSAFP	maternal serum alpha fetoprotein
multip	multiparous
MVU	Montevideo units
N/V	nausea/vomiting
neg	negative
NPO	nothing by mouth
NSAID	nonsteroidal anti-inflammatory drug
NST	nonstress test
NSVD	normal spontaneous vaginal delivery
NT	nontender
NTD	neural tube defect
nullip	nulliparous
OTC	over the counter
PE	physical exam
PGE 1	prostaglandin
pgy 1, 2, etc.	resident post graduate year 1, 2, 3, or 4

PIH	pregnancy-induced hypertension
pit	Pitocin
plt	platelet
PO	by mouth
POC	products of conception
pos	positive
PPD	purified protein derivative (test for TB)
PPH	postpartum hemorrhage
PPROM	preterm premature rupture of membranes
PR	by rectum
primip	primiparous
PRN	as needed
PROM	premature rupture of membranes
pt	patient
PTB/PTD	preterm birth/delivery
PTL	preterm labor
PV	per vagina
q	every
QD	one time per day
QHS	at hour of sleep
QID	four times per day
QOD	every other day
RDS	respiratory distress syndrome
RhoGam	Rh (D) immunoglobulin
r/o	rule out
ROM	rupture of membranes
ROS	review of systems
RR	respiratory rate
RRR	regular rate and rhythm
RTC/RTO	return to clinic/office
s/s	signs and symptoms

S>D	size greater than dates
S<D	size less than dates
SAB	spontaneous abortion
SOB	shortness of breath
SROM	spontaneous rupture of membranes
SSE	sterile speculum exam
STI	sexually transmitted infection
SVE	sterile vaginal exam
SX	surgery
TB	tuberculosis
TID	three times per day
TOC	test of cure
TVU	transvaginal ultrasound
tx	treatment
U	units
UCX	uterine contractions
UPI	uterine placental insufficiency
U/S	ultrasound
UTI	urinary tract infection
VBAC	vaginal birth after cesarean section
VS	vital signs
WNL	within normal limits

T P A L

T = Term deliveries ≥ 37 weeks

P = Preterm deliveries < 37 weeks

A = Abortion (elective or spontaneous) > 20 weeks

L = Living children

Name	Contact info	Address/Notes
Labor & Delivery		
Rapid Response Team/Code		
Postpartum		
Antepartum		
Peds		
Anesthesia		
Blood Bank		
Rx		
Respiratory		
Nurse Manager		
Dietary		
House keeping		
Laundry		
Social Work		

Locker combo:

Name	Contact info	Address/Notes
	Cell:	
	Office:	
Glove Size:	Home:	
	Cell:	
	Office:	
Glove Size:	Home:	
	Cell:	
	Office:	
Glove Size:	Home:	
	Cell:	
	Office:	
Glove Size:	Home:	
	Cell:	
	Office:	
Glove Size:	Home:	
	Cell:	
	Office:	
Glove Size:	Home:	
	Cell:	
	Office:	
Glove Size:	Home:	

Name	Contact info	Address/Notes
	Cell:	
	Office:	
Glove Size:	Home:	
	Cell:	
	Office:	
Glove Size:	Home:	
	Cell:	
	Office:	
Glove Size:	Home:	
	Cell:	
	Office:	
Glove Size:	Home:	
	Cell:	
	Office:	
Glove Size:	Home:	
	Cell:	
	Office:	
Glove Size:	Home:	
	Cell:	
	Office:	
Glove Size:	Home:	

NOTES

Index